Complete Party Planner

Also by Annabel Karmel

SuperFoods
Top 100 Baby Purees
Favorite Family Meals
The Healthy Baby Meal Planner

Complete Party Planner

Over 120 delicious recipes and party ideas for every occasion

Annabel Karmel

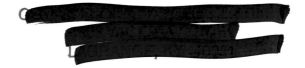

ATRIA BOOKS

NEW YORK   LONDON   TORONTO   SYDNEY

To my children, Nicholas, Lara, and Scarlett, who uncomplainingly ate their way through all the birthday cakes, gelatins, and chocolate cookies in this book yet surprisingly still managed to demolish all the leftover sweets from the photo shoots.

ATRIA BOOKS
1230 Avenue of the Americas
New York, NY 10020

A previous edition of this book was published in Great Britain in 2000 by Ebury Press

Karmel, Annabel.
Library of Congress Cataloging-in-Publication Data

    Complete party planner : over 120 delicious recipes and party ideas for every occasion / Annabel Karmel.
      p. cm.
    1. Entertaining. 2. Parties. 3. Cookery. I. Title.
TX731.K34 2006
793.2—dc22   2006045088

ISBN-13: 978-0-7432-9713-4
ISBN-10:   0-7432-9713-X

First Atria Books hardcover edition October 2006

10 9 8 7 6 5 4 3 2

For information about special discounts for bulk purchases,
please contact Simon & Schuster Special Sales:
1-800-456-6798 or business@simonandschuster.com.

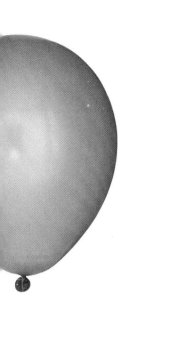

Contents

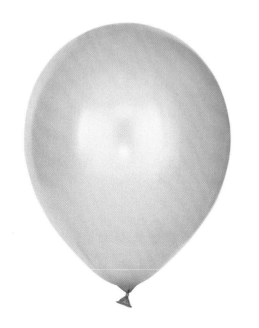

Introduction

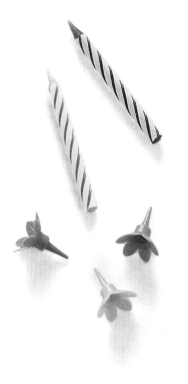

This is a book for everyone who has something to celebrate, and my aim is to make sure that your child's party goes with a swing. Whether it is a first-birthday celebration or you are looking for new ideas and inspiration to come up with something truly memorable after many years of organizing children's parties, there is something in this book for you. As a mother of three children, I have learned a lot from my own successes and failures. I remember my daughter showing the first signs of chicken pox and breaking out in angry red spots just as her friends were arriving for a party. Or there was the ill-fated disco party I organized where none of the children wanted to dance, and my son's sports party in the pouring rain where it was so muddy it took some skill just to remain upright. Yet sometimes the unexpected can make the day, and I overheard one boy tell his dad as he was leaving that he wanted a sports party on his birthday but only if it was raining. It turned out that the boys had more fun sliding around and getting caked in mud than if the sun had been shining!

Parental involvement means far more to your child than spending money on a lavish party. The smile on his or her face mirrors the love you show for your child. Be a part of their fun, don't sit on the sidelines, join in with their growing up—it's such fun. One of the most successful parties I gave

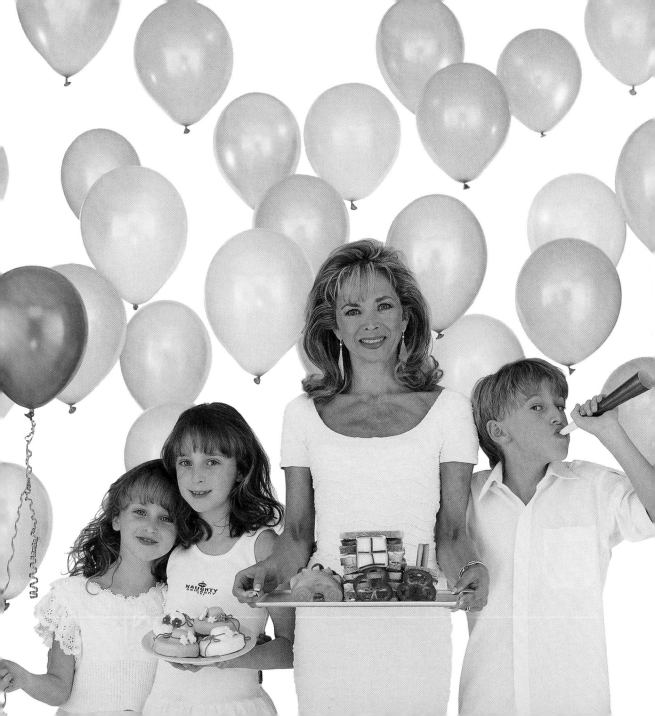

my son was a soccer party, and the highlight was inviting all the dads to play a game at the end against the boys. Despite the dads not having played soccer in at least twenty years, I've never seen a more competitive bunch. Needless to say, the boys loved every minute of it, but I think a lot of the dads suffered later on in the day!

Advance planning and organization are the secrets to success, and party preparation is all part of the fun. Once your child is old enough, he or she will enjoy being involved in helping to make the party invitations, choosing the games, or helping prepare the food, and this book is packed full of fun activities for you to share with your child.

An approaching birthday is the biggest event in a child's life, and although the charm for us wears off around the age of thirty-five, children look forward to it all year, counting the weeks to the special day with feverish excitement. Active participation is definitely a key to success. For my older daughter I organized a cooking party where—horror of horrors—no food was prepared in advance and it was up to the children to make their own. They had enormous fun rolling out dough, cutting out cookies, and making milkshakes. Yes, it was messy and you needed a team of willing helpers, but, boy, was it worth it to see their little faces beaming with pride at their

KEY FOR SYMBOLS
easy for children to help
N contains nuts
❄ suitable for freezing

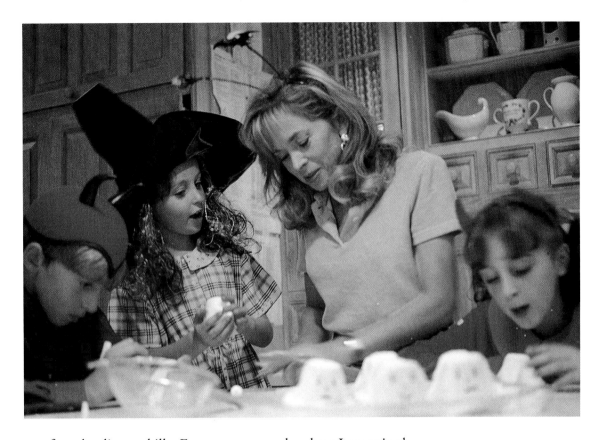

newfound culinary skills. For my younger daughter I organized
a beauty and jewelry-making party where the girls' faces and
hair were done, their nails painted, and before-and-after pictures
taken. In between, the budding supermodels also had the chance
to make jewelry and play party games.

From the original and fun invitation that sets the mood to the
last crumb of the novelty birthday cake, I hope that this book
will help ensure that your child's party is truly memorable.

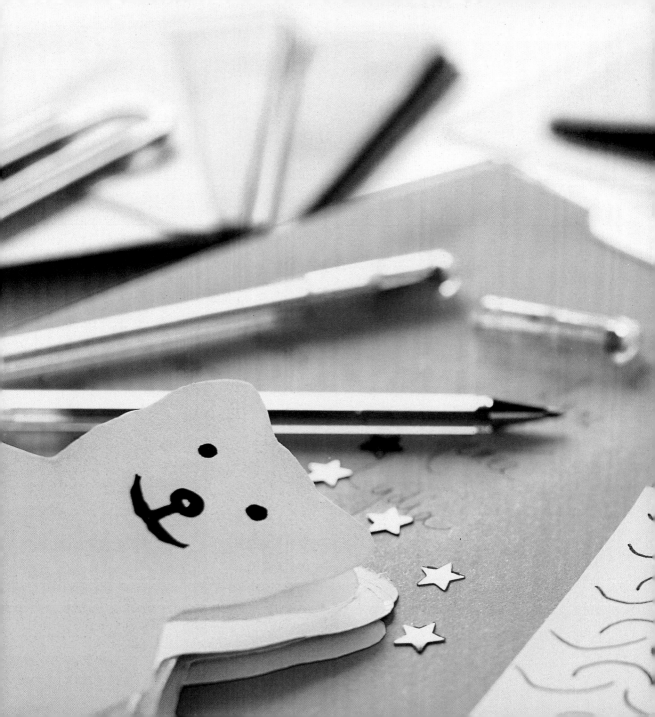

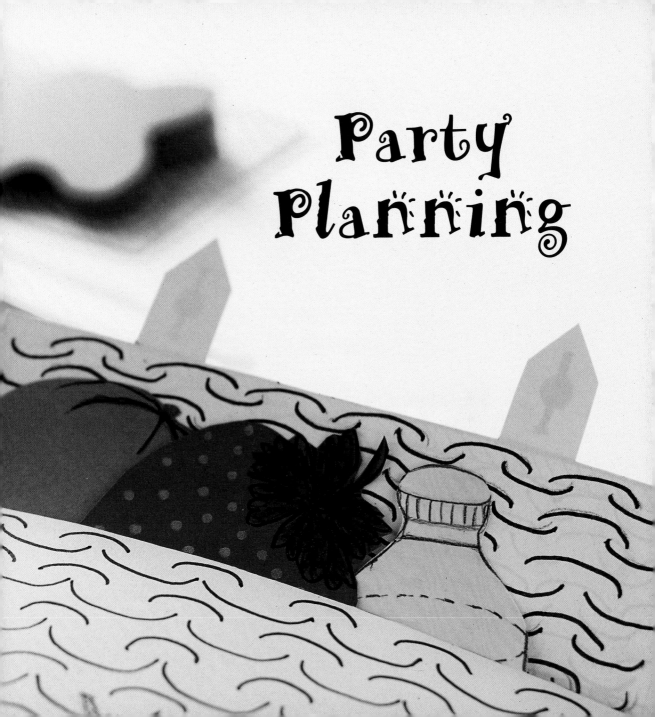

Party Planning

Planning Your Party

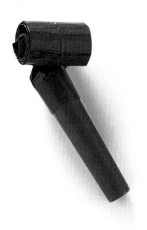

I always think that there is something quite personal about having a party at home, but it does involve quite a lot of organizing. You will probably need to move some of the furniture so there is enough room for the children to play games, and if there are a lot of children, you may need to rent tables and chairs. But if the thought of a whole bunch of excited kids running amok in your house fills you with dread, the answer might be to hold your party somewhere else.

Think about where you would like to hold the party in plenty of time, as some venues may need to be booked months in advance. Some ideas for possible venues include a local church hall, a school hall, an indoor gymnasium, and the local park. Other venues such as a skating rink, swimming pool, soccer field, museum, zoo, theme park, circus, theater or cinema, waterslide park, or a junior go-kart track will determine the theme of the party.

Involving Your Child

Whatever you choose to do, involve your child in the decision making and party preparation. Birthday parties are a big event in a child's life, and it is really important that your child be included in this way. There are many

Tip

For little children of two and under, invite parents along as well. Toddlers need more attention than one or two adults can give. At this age they won't need organized games, so have lots of toys for them to play with.

things that your child can be involved in, perhaps drawing a picture for the invitations, which you can then photocopy, or choosing the kind of games to be played. Sharing the party planning with you will be very exciting for your child and give him or her an enormous sense of importance—quite right and proper for the big day, after all.

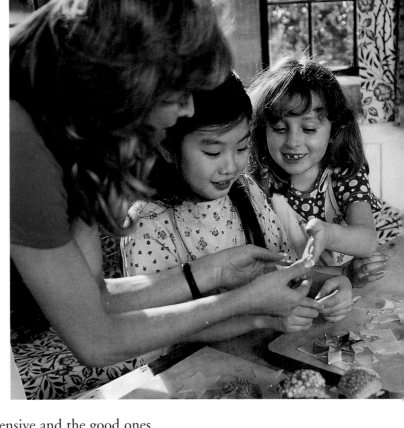

Entertainment

Children's party entertainers tend to be very popular, but they are expensive and the good ones will need to be booked well in advance. Of course, it makes life much easier to let the entertainer organize the entertainment for you, but in my experience, nothing will delight your child more than your efforts and the time you put in to make sure the party goes with a swing. There is such a fantastic variety of party games for all ages, and I find that children want to take part rather than be spectators. Don't make the party too long—two to two and a half hours is just about right.

Tip

If planning an outdoor party, do not assume the weather will be good. Have an alternative indoor venue that is close by.

The Party Countdown

8 weeks ahead
Book the venue and entertainer
(if appropriate).

4 weeks ahead
Decide on how many children you want
to invite and make a guest list with the
help of your child.
Decide on the theme or entertainment.
Make and send invitations.
Organize costumes (if appropriate).
Decide on your helpers, who may
be parents, relatives, or friends.
Rent tables and chairs (if necessary).

1 week ahead
Buy paper plates, cups, napkins,
balloons, candles, cake board.
Buy decorations, like banners
and streamers.
Plan the games, buy any special props,
and make a list.
Choose the music: Each age group has
their favorite music from nursery rhymes
for very young children to the latest pop
songs for older children.
Buy nonperishable ingredients for the
food.
Buy going-home presents (if necessary)
and prizes and wrap them.
Make a list of food for the party. Spread
the food preparation over several days
and make any party food that you want
to freeze in the week before the party.

2 days ahead

Call any RSVPs who have not responded.
Draw up the final guest list.
Shop for the remaining food for
the party.
Baking day: Bake the birthday cake and
make the cakes and cookies.
Make up the party bags (if necessary).
Sort out party clothes.
Check your camera and make sure you
have spare batteries.
Make sure you have candles and matches
for the cake.

1 day ahead

Decorate the cake.
Prepare gelatins and any other party
food that would be fine prepared the
day ahead.
Decorate the house and table.
Prepare the games.

Day of the party

Make the fresh party food such as
sandwiches, fresh fruit, etc. Keep
sandwiches fresh by covering them with
a damp cloth like a clean kitchen towel.
Blow up the balloons or buy some
helium-filled balloons.
If holding the party at home, decorate
the front door with balloons and maybe
a banner saying HAPPY BIRTHDAY.
Put a sign on the bathroom door and
lock rooms that are out of bounds.
Set the table and lay out the food.

Tips

Keep a first-aid kit on hand at the party in case of
accidents.
Do not give peanuts to children under the age of
three.

Making Invitations

A few examples are given here and then more specific ideas scattered through the book to tie in with the themed party ideas. See the following invitations, which will give you ideas for other ways to make your own:

Cooking Party on page 38

Sports Party on page 44

Makeup and Jewelry Party on page 80

Easter on page 120

Teddy Bears' Picnic on page 138

Fourth of July on page 147

Halloween on page 164

Christmas on page 188

An original handmade invitation will set the scene for a very special party. Making your own invitations can be a lot of fun, too, but keep your design quite simple, as you will need to make it several times. If possible, get your child involved in helping to make the invitations.

Jigsaw Invitation

You will need: store-bought, hand-drawn and photocopied, or computer-generated invitations. Write out all the details on the invitations or print them on the computer. Then cut the invitation into lots of pieces like a jigsaw puzzle. Put in a little note to say something like "Let's get together" and send to each of the guests.

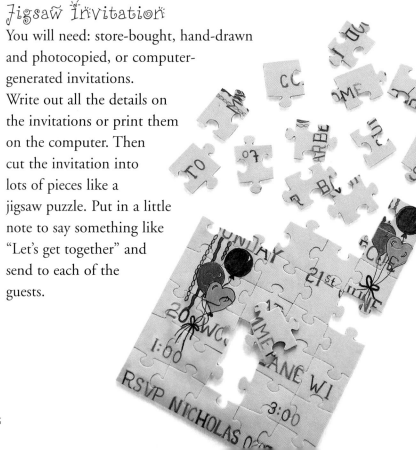

Baby Photo Invitation

You will need: cute photograph of the birthday girl or boy as a baby, balloons, permanent black marker pen. Photocopy the baby photo on a color photocopier and write on the front something like "Guess Who's Having a Birthday Party!" and add the party details on the back.

Balloon Invitation

Inflate a balloon but do not tie it. Ask someone to hold it for you and write the party details on the surface of the balloon using a permanent felt-tip pen, allow to dry, then let out the air. Place the balloon in an envelope with a note instructing the guest to blow up the balloon.

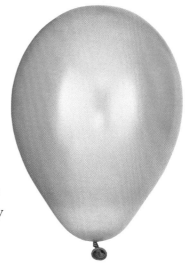

Party Games

Pick party games that are right for your child's age. They should be challenging but not too difficult. Have some inexpensive prizes on hand for the winners and try to make sure that everyone has a chance to win a prize. The first half hour of a party can be awkward, especially if some of the children don't know one another, so it is good to get them involved right from the start in some games to break the ice. Messy games like the Egyptian Mummy (see page 21) are best reserved for the end of the party.

Icebreakers

Paper Bag Mystery
Props: paper bags, mystery objects, twist ties. Label paper bags with each letter of your child's name and put objects that start with the corresponding letter into each of the bags and tie them at the top. The children have to guess what is in each of the bags by feeling the outside of the bag.

The Power of Advertising
Props: old magazines, scissors, pencils and paper.
Cut out illustrations or photographs advertising products from magazines, but make sure the product is not shown or named. Pin them all over the house before the children arrive. When they take off their coats, give each of the children a piece of paper and a pencil. The children then have to try to write down what the products are.

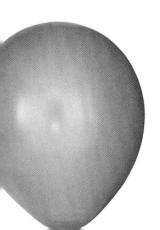

Ten minutes after the last guest has arrived, collect all the lists—whoever has identified the most products is the winner.

Hidden Stars

Props: packets of small colored stars.

Hide the stars around the room before the party. How well hidden they are will really depend on the children's age. The aim is for the children to find as many pairs of the same colored stars as they can. This could also be played with mini M&M's.

Hunt the Ping-Pong Balls

Props: Ping-Pong balls, permanent black marker pen.

Give guests a Ping-Pong ball with their name on it when they arrive and send them off one by one to another room to hide it. When the last guest has hidden the ball, it is time for all the guests to start looking for them. The guest whose ball is the last to be found is the winner.

Indoor Party Games

Musical Newspapers

Props: old newspapers.

Space out sheets of newspaper on the floor with one less than the number of children. Put on the music and the children can dance around. When the music stops, the children must leap onto a sheet of newspaper, and the child who doesn't find one is out. Remove a piece and start again, until there is only one person left. The same game can be played with pillows.

Memory Game

Props: a tray, various objects, pencils and paper.

Put a tray of objects in front of the children and give them two minutes in which to memorize the items. The older the children are, the more items you can put on the tray. Remove the tray and the children must write down on a piece of paper as many of the objects as they can remember.

Jelly Bean Hunt
Props: jelly beans.

Assign a point value to each color of jelly bean. The highest value goes to the color with the fewest number of beans. Hide the beans in the party room so they are in sight but well camouflaged. Set a time limit, at the end of which the child with the most points is the winner.

Hoop-la
Props: empty milk bottles, six hoops.

Arrange a collection of empty milk bottles on bits of paper with a score written on each. Get some hoops or cut out hoops from strong cardboard and give each child six. The children stand behind a line and throw hoops at the bottles. If the hoops go right over, the children score the number of points on the pieces of paper on which the hoops land.

Eat the Chocolate
Props: a very large bar of chocolate, plastic plate, knife and fork, dice, hat, scarf, pair of gloves, sunglasses.

The children sit in a circle and take turns throwing the dice. Anyone who throws a six leaps up, puts on all the clothes, and then has to try and cut and eat as much chocolate as possible until someone else throws a six. Sometimes a six is thrown even before the child manages to get all the clothes on, so you have to be quick. The winner is the child who eats the most chocolate.

Jumping Balloon Race
Props: two balloons.

Line up two teams at one end of a room behind a line. Give the person at the front of each team a balloon, which they should hold between their knees. On the given signal, the leaders race to the end of the room and back, jumping with the balloon between their knees. The balloon is given to each of the next players in turn and the winner is the team whose last player first arrives behind the line with the balloon. If the balloon floats away, then whoever let it go must return to the start line and begin again.

The Egyptian Mummy

Props: rolls of toilet paper.

Divide the children into teams and choose one "mummy" from each team (they should be about the same size) and give each mummy a roll of toilet paper. The mummies stand facing their teams with their legs together and arms by their sides. On "Go!" the first in each team runs up to their mummy and starts to bandage with the toilet paper, starting at the feet and

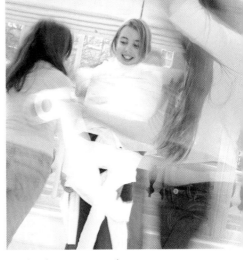

working upward. After about thirty seconds, the second player runs up and takes over and so on. If the paper tears, it must be tucked neatly into the folds before starting again. The winning team is the one that most successfully covers the mummy in a given time. The next prize is for the mummy who can divest himself or herself of the wrappings the quickest.

Bomb Squad

Prop: kitchen timer with a ticking sound.

Have the children leave the room. Set the timer for three minutes. Hide it but make sure the ticking sound is still audible. Have the children return to the room and tell them that their job is to listen for the "bomb" and find it before it goes off in three minutes. As the seconds tick by, the suspense will build up. If the children are quite successful at locating the "bomb," you can make it more challenging by setting the timer for two minutes or even just one.

Siamese Twins

Props: tennis balls.

Divide the children into two teams of even numbers and get them to stand at one end of the room. The first and second players hold hands and face each other, and a tennis ball is put between their foreheads. They have to run to the far end of the room and back without dropping the ball. If the ball drops, they have to go back and start again. When the first couple successfully returns, they place the ball between the second pair's foreheads, and so on until everyone in the team has had a go. If you want the game to last longer, you could allow each pair two turns.

Fishing Game

Props: old newspapers, scissors, yarn.

Cut out fish from newspaper and thread lengths of yarn through their heads. Players tie the yarn around their waists so that the fish are just trailing on the floor behind them. On "Go!," everyone has to try and catch the others' fish by stamping on them, but at the same time they must keep their own fish intact. The last one to keep his or her fish on the "line" is the winner.

Blindman's Buff

Prop: a dark scarf to make a good blindfold.

One of the guests volunteers to be blindfolded and is then turned around several times until disoriented. The other players move around quietly in a fairly small area and the blindfolded player has to try and catch one of them. It is a good idea to first remove any objects from the room that you think might get broken. Once caught, the player then has to stand still while the blindfolded child feels his or her face and body and tries to guess who is the captive. If the guess is correct, the two change places and the game starts again.

Paper Fashion Show

Props: newspaper, cellophane tape, scissors, string or ribbon, and whatever odds and ends you can find, like leftover wrapping paper or wallpaper.

Divide the children into pairs and put all the props on a table. One of each pair has to make an outfit for the partner to wear—give them a time limit of about fifteen minutes. Then hold a fashion show so that everyone can vote, giving marks out of ten for each outfit. But no one is allowed to vote for his or her own outfit.

Guess Whose Feet

Props: pen and paper, large sheet.

Divide the guests into two teams and send one team out of the room. The other team takes off their shoes and socks and lies down on the floor in a straight row. Drape a sheet over them so that only their feet are sticking out and put a piece of paper with a number on it next to each pair of feet. Tell the children to be very quiet and as still as possible and then bring the other team into the room. The members of this team then have to make a list of who they think the feet belong to. When they have chosen, remove the sheet and reveal the children's identities. Repeat with the second team. The team with the most correct answers wins.

Famous People

Props: pencils and paper.

Make up a chart of anagrams made up of famous people's names. Give each child pencil and paper and see how many names they can work out in a given time.

Pass the Parcel (with a twist)

Props: one large prize, various small prizes, newspaper, pen and paper.

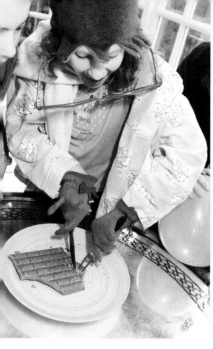

Choose one big prize and lots of little prizes like candies, pencils, erasers, hair ornaments. Also write several forfeits on pieces of paper like "Sing a song" or "Stand on your head." First wrap the main prize in newspaper, then continue to wrap in more layers of newspaper and in each layer choose to put either a small prize or forfeit. Arrange the children in a circle, start the music, and get them to pass the parcel around the circle. When the music stops, the child holding the parcel has to unwrap one layer, enjoying the forfeit or prize accordingly. Continue until someone gets to unwrap the main prize. Whoever is controlling the music should make sure that everyone in the circle gets a turn to unwrap the parcel.

Ambidextrous Skills

Props: pen, paper, pencils, hat.
Have the same number of pieces of paper as guests and on each write the name of an object such as a chair or a television. Put the pieces of paper in a hat and choose one of the children to take out a piece of paper and then draw the object with the wrong hand. Whoever guesses correctly what the child has drawn is next.

Sucking M&M's

Props: straws, M&M's, bowl, and plate.
Have a pile of M&M's on a plate, and an empty bowl. The object of the game is to get as many M&M's as possible into the bowl by sucking them onto the end of a straw and then letting them drop into the bowl. Use a new straw for each competitor. The one to transfer the most M&M's in a set time is the winner.

Outdoor Party Games

Wheelbarrow Race

This is a fun game for outdoors on a lawn. Everyone chooses a partner. The children take turns being the wheelbarrow and walk on their hands while the other child holds their ankles. For an even more difficult game, you can attempt to do this backward.

Sack Race

Props: black trash bags.

Everyone climbs into a "sack," or black trash bag. On "Go!," the children jump along with both feet in the sack. The first one to cross the finish line without falling over is the winner.

Spud and Spoon Race

Props: large spoons and potatoes.

On "Go!," the children have to run to the finish line balancing a potato on a spoon. If the potato falls off, they must pick it up with the spoon as fast as possible, without touching it with their fingers, and begin again.

Crab Race

Line up teams at one end of the lawn (or room) and show them how to grasp their ankles and run sideways like a crab. The first member of each team has to go to the far end of the lawn and back and then the second member of the team can go and so on. The winning team is the one whose last member gets back to base first. Any children who let go of their ankles or fall over have to start all over again.

Up and Under

Form the teams into lines and space each member about two feet apart. The child at the back leapfrogs over the one in front, crawls between the legs of the next player, leapfrogs over the third, and so on. As soon as a player has been jumped over or crawled under, he or she has to move back a place. As soon as the first team member has completed the line, the next player has a turn. The first team back in their original positions is the winning team.

Dressing-Up Race

Props: 2 hats, 2 shirts, 2 pairs of trousers, 2 pairs of sunglasses, 2 pairs of boots. This is a relay race with a difference for two teams. Have a hat, shirt, trousers, sunglasses, and boots laid out at equally spaced intervals on the way to the finish line. The players must run to the clothes and put them on as they come to them, then run to the finish line, touch it, and race back again removing the clothes in reverse order, thereby leaving them in the correct place for the next player. Each player completes the course and the team that finishes first is the winner.

Nature Scavenger Hunt

Make a list of things to find in nature, such as a pinecone, daisy, leaf. Give a copy of the list to each child and set a time limit. The child who manages to gather the most objects or the team with the most objects is the winner.

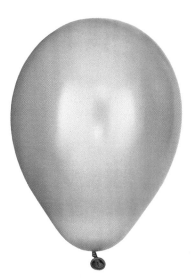

Prizes and Going-Away Bags

After the party, children expect to go home with a party bag full of favors. Set a limit to how much you wish to spend. Here are some of the things you could buy for party bags. Your child will love helping to make up these bags, and from experience I have found it is best that everyone gets the same. However, boys and girls will have different favors. You could also wrap up a slice of birthday cake in foil and pop it in the bag, too.

Pens, pencils, erasers, sharpeners, notebooks
Stickers
Hair ornaments
Jewelry
Light-stick necklace
Nail polish
Bead kits
Bubble bath
Packets of seeds
Bubble kits
Marzipan animals

Yo-yos
Coloring books
Mini collage kit
Paper airplanes
Badges
Miniature bouncy balls
Silly Putty
Mini magic trick

For prizes, put some of these into a hat and have a lucky dip. If it is a mixed party, have a lucky dip each for girls and boys.

If there are lots of presents for the birthday boy or girl, I know that with my own children I usually allow them to open some after the party and then open one or two a day after that. It is something to look forward to after school. Don't forget to make a list of the presents that everyone has given so that your child can send thank-you notes.

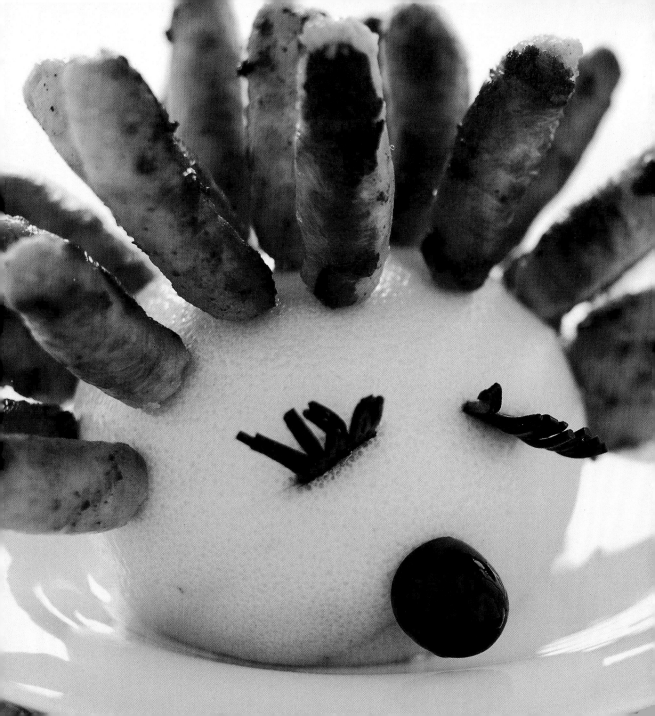

Savory Party Food

Bashful Sausage Hedgehog

SERVES 8

Licorice laces
1 large grapefruit
1 large black olive, pitted
Toothpicks
Brown and serve breakfast
  sausages

This is quick and easy to assemble and looks great—the sausages will vanish in no time at all.

To make the hedgehog's eyelashes, curl short lengths of licorice by wrapping them around a pencil and securing with tightly wrapped foil. Set the eyelashes aside for 30 minutes to take shape.

CUT A THIN SLICE off the base of the grapefruit so that it sits flat, then, using a sharp knife, make two slits for the eyes and insert the licorice eyelashes. To form the hedgehog's nose, attach the olive to the grapefruit using half a toothpick.

COOK THE SAUSAGES, spear with toothpicks, and stick into the grapefruit to form the hedgehog's spines.

OVERLEAF: Bashful Sausage Hedgehog

Avocado Frog Dip

You can decorate this tasty and nutritious dip with slices of cucumber and egg and stuffed olives for the eyes and strips of chives for the mouth. I like to serve it with a selection of raw vegetables and cheese cut into novelty shapes using cookie cutters.

Cut the avocado in half, remove the pit, and scoop out the flesh. Mash or blend together all the ingredients, seasoning lightly with salt and pepper and perhaps a few drops of Tabasco sauce. Decorate to look like a frog.

SERVES 6

1 large ripe avocado
1½ teaspoons lemon juice
2 tablespoons cream cheese
1 tablespoon snipped chives or
    finely chopped scallions
1 tomato, peeled, seeded,
    and chopped
Salt and freshly ground black
    pepper
Tabasco sauce (optional)

DECORATION
  2 slices cucumber
    2 slices hard-boiled egg
    2 stuffed olives
    2 chives or scallions
    Cheese and vegetable
    cutouts

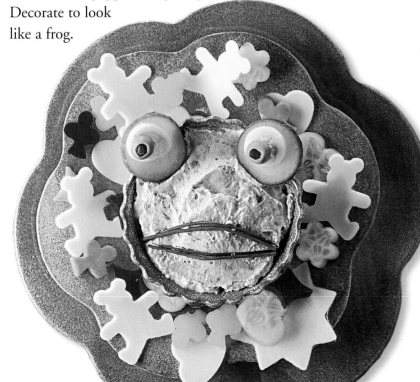

31

Crudités with Annabel's Dip

SERVES 8

DIP

½ cup finely chopped onion

½ cup canola oil

¼ cup rice wine vinegar

3 tablespoons water

1 tablespoon chopped fresh
   gingerroot

2 tablespoons chopped celery

2 tablespoons soy sauce

3 teaspoons tomato paste

3 teaspoons sugar

2 teaspoons lemon juice

Salt and freshly ground black
   pepper

This dip is one of my children's favorite things to eat. They love it as a snack when they come home from school and it's been a great way to get them to enjoy eating vegetables. As well as colorful vegetable sticks for a party, you could also serve bread sticks or you can use mini cutters to cut larger vegetables like red peppers or fat carrots into shapes like small stars. The dip also makes a delicious salad dressing.

To make the dip, combine all the ingredients in a blender or food processor and process until smooth.

FOR THE CRUDITÉS, chop into sticks or convenient sizes any or all of the following vegetables: carrot, cucumber, bell pepper, celery, lettuce, cherry tomatoes, sugar snap peas, and cauliflower florets. Arrange the vegetables on a plate with the dip served in a bowl in the center of the plate.

Hot Potato Wedges with Sour Cream Dip

Children love eating things that they can pick up with their fingers and dip into a sauce.

Preheat the oven to 400°F. Cut each potato into about six wedges. Place the potatoes in a roasting pan. Add the olive oil, toss, and sprinkle with the paprika and salt and bake for 35 to 40 minutes, turning a few times.

TO MAKE THE DIP, simply mix together all the ingredients. It's best to make the dip the day before or at least several hours ahead to allow time for all the flavors to blend.

SERVES 4

POTATO WEDGES

3 medium potatoes (Yukon gold potatoes are good for this)

1 tablespoon olive oil

½ teaspoon paprika

½ teaspoon salt

SOUR CREAM DIP

½ cup sour cream or crème fraîche

1 tablespoon light cream

1 teaspoon lemon juice

1 tablespoon snipped chives

Salt and freshly ground black pepper

OVERLEAF: Cheese Wands (page 40), Sausage Airplanes (page 36), Magic Toadstools (page 36), Hot Potato Wedges with Sour Cream Dip (this page)

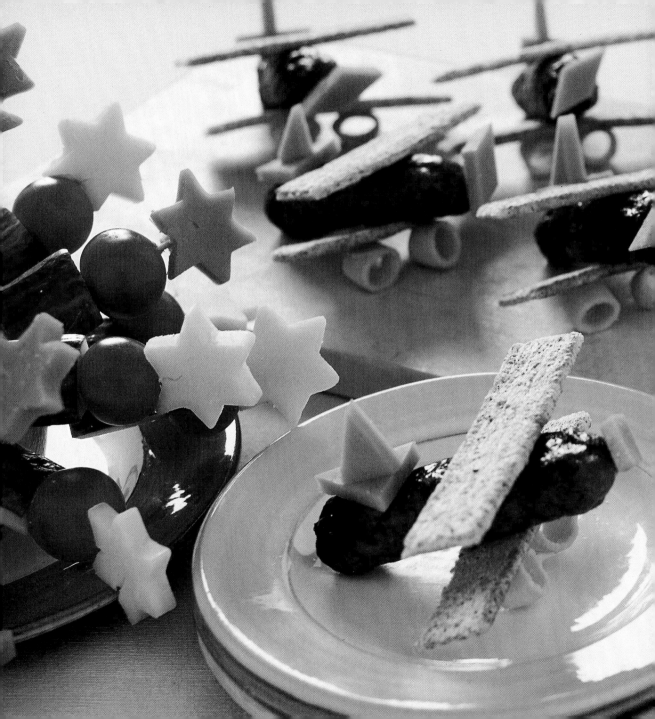

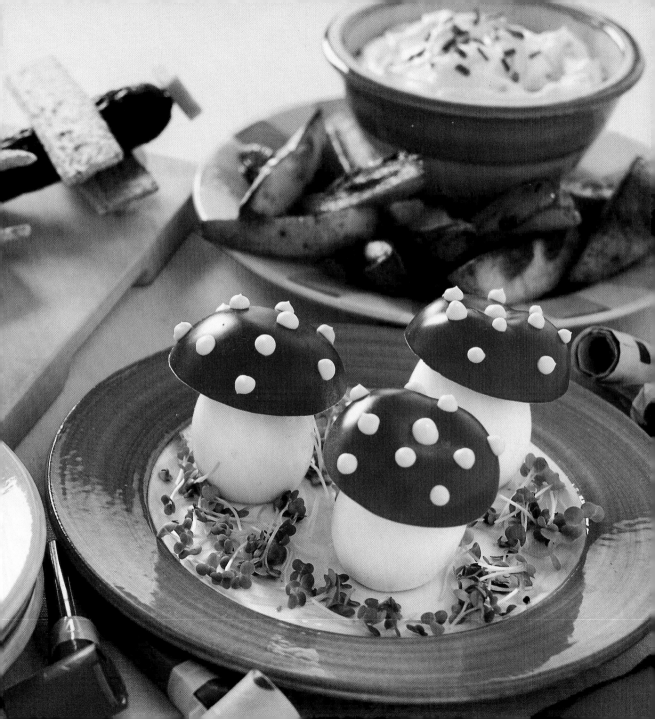

Sausage Airplanes

MAKES 6 AIRPLANES

6 chicken sausages

12 Combos crackers

12 long, thin crispbreads

Cheese spread, such as Cheez Whiz

6 diamonds and 12 triangles cheese cut from Cheddar or Gruyère

Watch that these sausages don't take off before you manage to grab them!

Grill the sausages. Attach two empty Combos to six of the crispbreads using a little of the cheese spread as "glue," to form the wheels of the planes. Rest the cooked sausages over the crispbreads. Position a second crispbread on top of each sausage and secure with cheese spread to form the other wing. Attach a diamond of cheese for the propeller using the cheese spread and form the tail of the plane with two triangles of cheese.

Magic Toadstools

MAKES 6 TOADSTOOLS

6 hard-boiled eggs

Cheese spread, such as Cheez Whiz

3 small tomatoes, halved

Alfalfa sprouts

These are easy to prepare, look fabulous, and are made with healthy ingredients.

Trim the top and bottom of each of the hard-boiled eggs so that they are flat and arrange on a plate. Squeeze or pipe dots of cheese spread over the tomatoes and place a halved tomato on top of each of the boiled eggs. Decorate the plate with alfalfa sprouts.

Pizza Faces

These make popular party food and it is a lot of fun to let the children choose the toppings themselves before the pizzas are baked in the oven. It is also fun to decorate the pizzas to look like faces. As a quick alternative, you can use ready-made pizza dough, split toasted English muffins, kaiser rolls, or bagels for the pizza bases and a ready-made tomato sauce.

Sift the flour and salt into a bowl and rub in the butter using your fingertips until the mixture resembles fine bread crumbs. Stir in the cheese and then mix in the milk to form a soft dough. Roll out on a lightly floured work surface to a thickness of about ¼ inch and cut out 10 mini pizzas using a 3-inch cutter.

TO MAKE THE TOMATO SAUCE, melt the butter in a pan, add the onion, and sauté for about 4 minutes until soft. Stir in the drained tomatoes, tomato paste, Italian seasoning, and salt and pepper to taste. Bring to a simmer and cook for about 2 minutes until slightly thickened.

PREHEAT THE OVEN to 425°F. Top each pizza with a heaping tablespoon of the tomato sauce. Add a few slices of mushrooms, top with a slice of tomato, some corn, and some of the grated mozzarella. Drizzle some olive oil on top. Lay the pizzas on a greased baking pan and bake for about 18 minutes.

MAKES 10 MINI PIZZAS

1½ cups self-rising flour

1 teaspoon salt

4 tablespoons unsalted butter

¾ cup grated sharp Cheddar cheese

½ cup milk

TOMATO SAUCE

1 tablespoon unsalted butter

1 small onion, finely chopped

One 14.5-ounce can diced tomatoes, drained

1 tablespoon tomato paste

¼ teaspoon Italian seasoning

Salt and freshly ground black pepper

3 sliced button mushrooms

2 tomatoes, sliced

⅔ cup canned or frozen corn

1 cup grated mozzarella cheese

1 tablespoon olive oil

Cooking Party

COOKING PARTY INVITATIONS
You will need: small wooden spoons, black permanent marker pen, 8½ x 11-inch sheets of colored construction paper, padded envelopes. On the handle of the wooden spoon write something like "Come to Lara's Cooking Party." Draw the outline of a rolling pin on colored paper, cut around the outline, and write on the rolling pin the details of the party. Place the rolling pin and wooden spoon inside a padded envelope. Either provide cheap aprons at the party or ask the children on the invitations to bring aprons with them.

Children adore cooking and you don't have to wait for a birthday to hold a cooking party. During school holidays, ask your child to invite some friends over and let them choose some favorite recipes to prepare. The children will have the most wonderful time making the dishes, together with a little adult supervision where necessary, and will be very proud to have prepared their own meal, which they might share with the parents if you get lucky.

The perfect age for a cooking party is between five and twelve years. However, if you intend it to be a birthday party and want to invite a number of children, you will really need quite a large kitchen. You may also need to rent or borrow some extra tables for the children to work on to prevent it from becoming a battleground. It will be important to have some adults to assist you in helping the children with their cooking and to do things like putting food in the oven or measuring ingredients.

There will also be a lot of cleaning up between recipes. So it is a good idea to have breaks in the cooking when the children can play party games in another room and your helpers can arrange the ingredients so that they are set up for the next recipe when the children come back to the kitchen.

Recipes

Plan the recipes with your child. Divide up the ingredients so that children can work in pairs and, where appropriate, measure ingredients beforehand and have them ready in small plastic bags or bowls. Have the instructions for each of the recipes printed out on separate pieces of paper in easy steps for the children to follow. Make a little book of recipes with a cover and staple together so that the children can take it home with them afterward. Before they attempt each recipe, read out the instructions and explain each step carefully to the children.

Once you have chosen the recipes and you know how many children are coming, make a list of all the utensils you will need, such as baking pans, mixing bowls, chopping boards, etc. Borrow some from friends, neighbors, relatives, or parents of the children coming to the party and pick them up a couple of days before the party.

Make sure that you take lots of photos, as this will be a very memorable party and there are bound to be some great action shots. It's great to see the children sit down and tuck into a meal that they have prepared themselves. You can pack up any extra food in individual boxes so that the children can take it home to their parents, who are bound to be very impressed!

IDEAL COOKING PARTY RECIPES
You will probably want to choose four of them.

Pizza Faces (page 37)

Cheese Wands (page 40)

Cheesy Feet and Hands (page 46)

Bagel Snake (page 53)

Chocolate Aliens (page 62)

Heart-Shaped Faces (page 66)

Coconut Kisses (page 69)

Apple Smiles (page 72)

Jam Tarts (page 88)

Buzzy Bees (page 89)

White Chocolate Rice Krispies Squares (page 90)

Any of the drinks on pages 96–97.

Mini Chicken Burgers

MAKES ABOUT 15 MINI BURGERS

4 boneless, skinless chicken
   breasts
2 medium onions, chopped
3 tablespoons ketchup
Salt and freshly ground black
   pepper
½ cup fine matzo meal or fine
   bread crumbs
Canola oil

These are easy to prepare and are especially good served with oven-baked fries and ketchup.

Cut the chicken into small pieces and put in a food processor with the onions. Chop for a few seconds. Transfer to a mixing bowl and stir in the ketchup, seasoning, and 2 tablespoons of the matzo meal. Using your hands, form the mixture into about 15 small burgers and coat with the remaining matzo meal. Heat the oil in a large frying pan and fry the burgers for 2 to 3 minutes on each side.

Cheese Wands

MAKES AS MANY AS YOU LIKE

1 large grapefruit
Variety of cheeses, such as
   Cheddar, Gruyère, Gouda
Cucumber
Cherry tomatoes
6-inch skewers

This is an appealing way to serve some healthy party food.

Cut the base off the grapefruit so that it is flat, cover with foil, and place in the center of a serving plate. Cut the cheese into ½-inch slices and then cut into star shapes using cookie cutters. Thread chunks of cucumber, cheese stars, and cherry tomatoes onto the skewers. Stick the skewers into the grapefruit so that it is evenly covered.

Chicken Nuggets with Potato Chips

I make these with cheese and onion chips, but you could try other flavors, too. These nuggets can be made in advance and then just heated through in the oven.

Cut each chicken breast into eight pieces and marinate in the lemon juice and garlic for about 30 minutes. Remove the chicken from the marinade, dip each piece first in the seasoned flour, then in the egg, and finally in a mixture of the bread crumbs and crushed chips. Heat the oil in a large frying pan, add the chicken pieces, and sauté for about 5 minutes, turning occasionally, until golden and cooked through.

MAKES 16 CHICKEN NUGGETS

2 large boneless, skinless
   chicken breasts
Juice of 1 small lemon
1 small clove garlic, thinly
   sliced
Flour seasoned with salt and
   freshly ground black pepper
1 large egg, lightly beaten
½ cup fresh white bread
   crumbs
½ cup crushed sour cream and
   onion chips
Canola oil

Cucumber Crocodile

SERVES 4 TO 6

1 carrot (optional)
1¼ cucumbers
Toothpicks
Variety of cheeses
Fresh pineapple, cut into
    chunks, or 1 small can
    pineapple chunks
2 cherry tomatoes

This looks amazing, it's great for parties, and it also makes a fabulous prop for your own children's healthy snacks. I like to use a variety of cheeses, but cubes of ham or chicken also work well in place of the cheese.

Cut a long strip from the carrot, if using, with a vegetable peeler. Cut this into a strip about ½ inch wide and cut along one side to form a serrated edge. These are the crocodile's teeth. Cut a wedge from one end of the whole cucumber to make the crocodile's mouth. Insert the carrot teeth, if using. Cut the quarter cucumber into two 1-inch-wide slices, cut these in half, and then shape into feet with a triangle cut out of them. Attach these to the whole cucumber using toothpicks cut in half. Cut the cheese into cubes. Thread cheese and pineapple cubes onto several toothpicks and spear the ends into the cucumber. Cut a toothpick in half and use the two halves to attach the cherry tomatoes to form the crocodile's eyes.

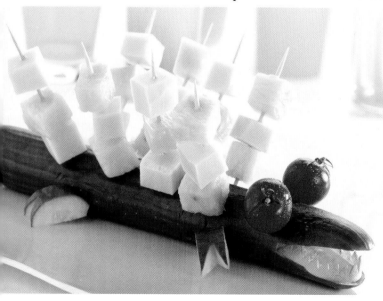

Mini Burgers

The apple in these burgers gives them a deliciously sweet taste and keeps them lovely and moist, too. You can serve them without the bun, but it's fun to use buns and pipe the first letter of the children's names on top of each.

Sauté the onion in the oil for 6 to 7 minutes until softened and then mix in all the other ingredients and form into about 12 small burgers. Shallow-fry or cook on a griddle. Cut the mini rolls in half, place the burgers on some lettuce, and top with the cheese stars, if using. Add some ketchup.

MAKES ABOUT 12 MINI BURGERS

❄

BURGERS

1 medium onion, finely chopped

1 tablespoon canola oil

1 pound ground beef or lamb

1 chicken bouillon cube dissolved in 2 tablespoons hot water

1 large apple, peeled and grated, excess juice squeezed out

½ beaten large egg

About 1 cup fresh bread crumbs (from 2 slices white bread, crusts removed)

1 tablespoon chopped fresh parsley

½ teaspoon hamburger or grill seasoning, such as McCormick's

Salt and freshly ground black pepper

FRYING

Canola oil for shallow-frying

SERVING

Mini rolls

Lettuce

Cheese slices cut into stars (optional)

Ketchup

Sports Party

SOCCER PARTY INVITATIONS
You will need: 8½ x 11-inch paper, pencils, crayons. Design the invitations to look like your son's or daughter's favorite soccer team's jersey. Draw a jersey on a sheet of paper and write the details of the party across the front. Photocopy as many as you need, then color in and cut out along the outline. The number could correspond to your child's age. It would be fun to send a reply card in the shape and design of a soccer ball.

This is the perfect party for a group of energetic boys or girls. Ideally, it should be an outdoor party, but a rented gym or large hall would be fine, too. Plan the party as outlined on pages 12–15.

When choosing the sporting events, be sure that you have a mixture of individual and team games. For the latter, it is best to divide the children into more, smaller teams so that the party doesn't become too competitive. Also, spread the talent among the teams so that they are pretty well balanced. Organize a timetable of events and organize all the equipment, such as a long ribbon for the finish line.

Teams can compete against each other in heats. For example, if there are twenty-four children, they can be divided into four teams of six. So two teams would compete against each other at a time and then the two winners of the teams would compete to find the overall winner. Award two points for the winner and one point for the runner-up. Consider holding an Olympic Games party and award "gold," "silver," and "bronze" medals to the amateur athletes.

44

Adding to the Fun

- For a soccer match, have a large board with the two teams written on them, calling each a color. Buy different-colored wide ribbon and tie a length around the arm of each player according to which team they are on.

- Organize some medals, prizes, or miniature silver cups for different categories, like best goalie, best striker, best dribbler, MVP, which can be handed out after the party.

Ideas for Sporting Events

4 x 100-meter relay race
Three-legged race
Obstacle course
Jumping Balloon Race (page 20)
Siamese Twins (page 22)
Wheelbarrow Race (page 25)
Spud and Spoon Race (page 25)
Crab Race (page 25)
Up and Under (page 26)
Dressing-Up Race (page 26)

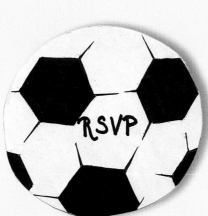

RSVP

Cheesy Feet and Hands

MAKES 4

4 tablespoons unsalted butter

One 8-ounce puff pastry sheet (frozen uncooked pastry sheet, thawed)

2 large eggs

2 cups grated cheese, such as Cheddar

Tomato puree or ketchup (optional)

You will need to make templates of feet and hands using a sheet of plastic or oak tag for the children to cut around. Alternatively, you could use cookie cutters (such as animal shapes) to cut out different cheese pastry shapes.

Grease a large baking pan with the butter and preheat the oven to 400°F. Sprinkle a clean work surface with a little flour and roll out the pastry with a rolling pin. Prick it with a fork to stop it from rising while it bakes. Place the feet and hand templates on the pastry and cut around them. Beat the eggs with a fork and brush over the pastry. Sprinkle with the cheese. Lift the feet and hands very carefully onto the baking pan. If you like, you can decorate the toenails and fingernails with a little tomato puree or ketchup. Bake for 10 to 15 minutes, then cool on a wire rack.

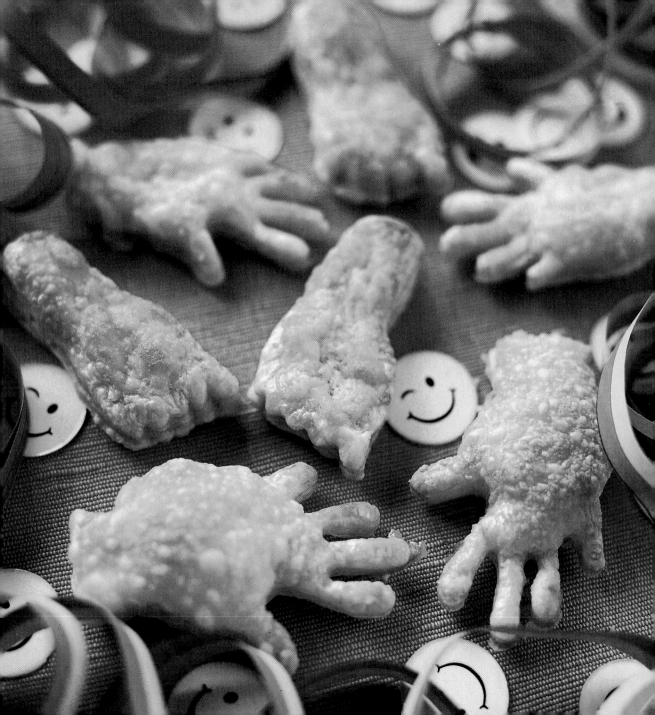

Sandwiches

🧑‍🍳 *Presentation is very important to a child, and fortunately sandwiches can come in many different shapes, sizes, and colors. There are many varieties of bread to choose from, such as raisin bread, pita bread pockets, bagels, and kaiser rolls. Here are some ideas to make sandwiches look extra special.*

NOVELTY-SHAPED SANDWICHES   Use cookie cutters to cut sandwiches into animal shapes, little people, cars, trains, etc. These sandwiches can be filled or open-face.

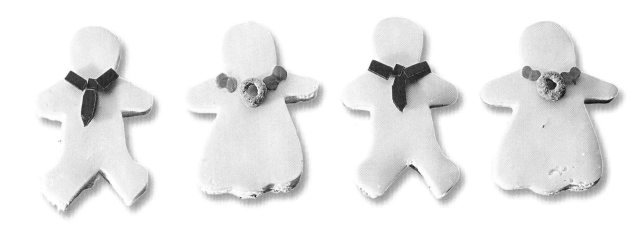

PINWHEEL SANDWICHES To make a pinwheel sandwich, choose a fairly dense bread and, if you can, chill it first, as it will then be easier to handle. Remove the crusts from two slices of bread, then place the slices on a board, with the shorter sides slightly overlapping, and roll them together with a rolling pin to join the slices together and to make the bread more pliable. Spread with a filling whose color contrasts with the color of the bread—something like smoked salmon and cream cheese mixed with a little ketchup, or peanut butter and strawberry jam. Roll up the bread like a jelly roll. Using a sharp knife, slice into wheels. If making ahead, wrap the roll tightly with plastic wrap and set aside in the fridge, and slice just before serving.

SPOTTY SANDWICHES To make spotty sandwiches, use the tip of a pastry bag to remove small circles from a slice of white and a slice of whole-wheat bread. Place the white bread discs in the holes in the whole-wheat bread and the whole-wheat discs in the holes in the white bread.

PITA BREAD POCKETS Warm a small pita bread in a toaster or preheated oven, cut in half, and fill with a savory filling such as strips of chicken or turkey, or salad or hummus.

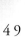

Peanut butter and strawberry
    jam
Mayonnaise and cucumber
Grated Cheddar cheese and
    ham
Swiss cheese and lettuce or
    cream cheese and tomato

DOUBLE-DECKER SANDWICHES Spread a slice of whole-wheat bread on both sides with butter and spread two slices of white bread on one side only. Choose one from a pair of fillings and spread it over one of the slices of white bread. Cover with the whole-wheat bread and spread it with the other filling. Put the second slice of white bread on top. Cut off the crusts, wrap in plastic wrap, and set aside in the fridge. To serve, cut into three strips and then cut each strip into three squares.

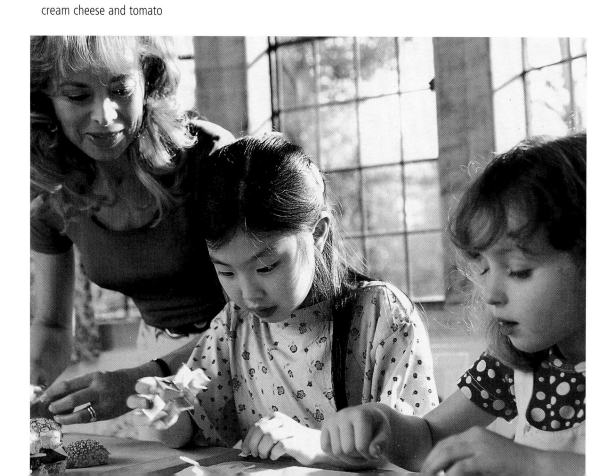

Great Sandwich Fillings

Chopped hard-boiled egg mashed with a little soft margarine or
butter and mayonnaise and sprinkled with shredded lettuce

Peanut butter and grape jelly

Cream cheese and cucumber

Peanut butter

Peanut butter, honey, and sliced banana

Nutella and banana

Peanut butter and strawberry jam

Grated Cheddar cheese and finely grated carrot mixed with a
little mayonnaise

Tuna or salmon salad with mayonnaise and chopped celery or
scallions

Grated Cheddar cheese and mango chutney

Chicken salad and shredded lettuce

Cream cheese with diced ham

Mashed sardines mixed with a little ketchup

Sliced Swiss cheese, tomato, and shredded lettuce

Taramasalata

Small cooked shrimp with mayonnaise or cocktail sauce
(see page 58) and shredded lettuce

Crisp bacon, lettuce, and tomato

Pastrami with a little mayonnaise and Dijon mustard
mixed together

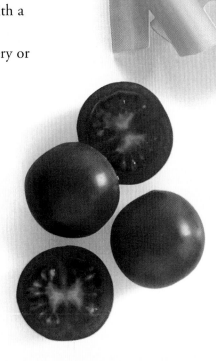

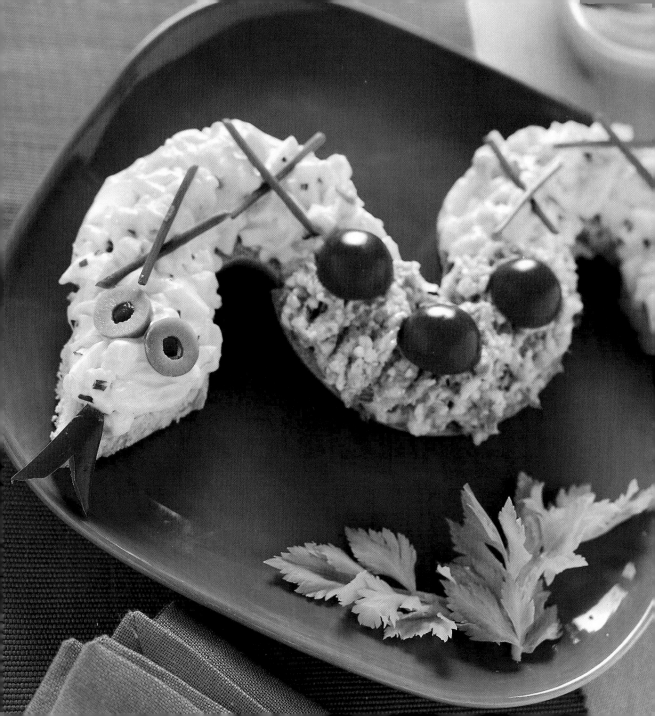

Bagel Snake

This is a fun way of arranging sandwiches, and I find that bagels are popular with both children and their moms and dads. You can make the snake as long as you like, depending on how many bagels you use, and you can use a variety of toppings. I have chosen tuna and egg toppings, which are both nutritious, but, of course, there are an infinite variety of ingredients that you could choose, such as cream cheese and cucumber.

Slice the bagels in half and then cut each half down the center to form a semicircle. Cut out the head of the snake from one of the pieces of bagel and the tail from another. Mix the ingredients for the tuna salad topping and mix the ingredients for the egg salad topping. Spread half the bagels with tuna and half with egg.

DECORATE THE TUNA TOPPING with halved cherry tomatoes and the egg topping with strips of chives arranged in a crisscross pattern. Arrange the bagels to form the body of a snake. Then attach the head to the snake's body and arrange two slices of stuffed olive to form the eyes and cut out a forked tongue from the strip of bell pepper.

2 bagels

TUNA SALAD TOPPING

One 6-ounce can tuna in olive oil, drained

2 tablespoons ketchup

2 tablespoons crème fraîche or plain yogurt

2 scallions, finely sliced

EGG SALAD TOPPING

2 or 3 hard-boiled Eggland's Best eggs, chopped

3 tablespoons mayonnaise

1 tablespoon snipped chives

Salt and freshly ground black pepper

DECORATION

Cherry tomatoes, halved

Chives

1 stuffed olive, sliced

Strip of red bell pepper

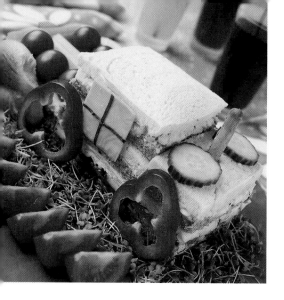

Tractor Sandwich

With a little imagination, assorted sandwiches can take on a whole new look.

This makes a great centerpiece for a birthday party and never fails to impress. Simply lay out different breads, spread with different but complementary fillings like those suggested, and form into the shape of a tractor. Make the wagon from 1½ bagels, and line up some fresh produce such as cherry tomatoes, cucumber, and celery. Make the wheels from sliced bell peppers and carrots, the windows from cheese slices and chives (these will stick better if heated for a few seconds in a microwave), and insert a sesame stick for the funnel. The children will have a great time taking it to pieces.

Slices of whole-wheat,
   multigrain, or white bread
Fillings such as egg and
   shredded lettuce, ham and
   cheese, and cream cheese,
   cucumber, and tomato
2 bagels
Cherry tomatoes
Celery
Red bell peppers, cored,
   seeded, and sliced
Carrots
Cheese slices
Chives
Sesame stick

Funny Fish Sandwich

It takes only a few minutes to transform a simple sandwich into a real showstopper!

Cut the roll open just below the middle and spread both halves with butter. Lay a few lettuce leaves on the bottom half, arrange some slices of egg on top, and spread with a little mayonnaise or cheese slices. Position two thick slices of tomato so that they protrude a little at one end. Cut a shallow groove along the center top of the roll and insert halved cucumber slices to look like fins. Place this on top of the bottom half of the roll and secure two blueberries with toothpicks to make the eyes.

MAKES 1 FISH SANDWICH

1 hot dog roll

Butter

Soft lettuce leaves, such as
   Boston

Hard-boiled egg

Mayonnaise or cheese slices

1 tomato, sliced

Cucumber slices

2 blueberries

Toothpicks

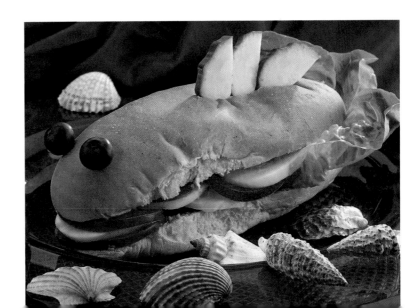

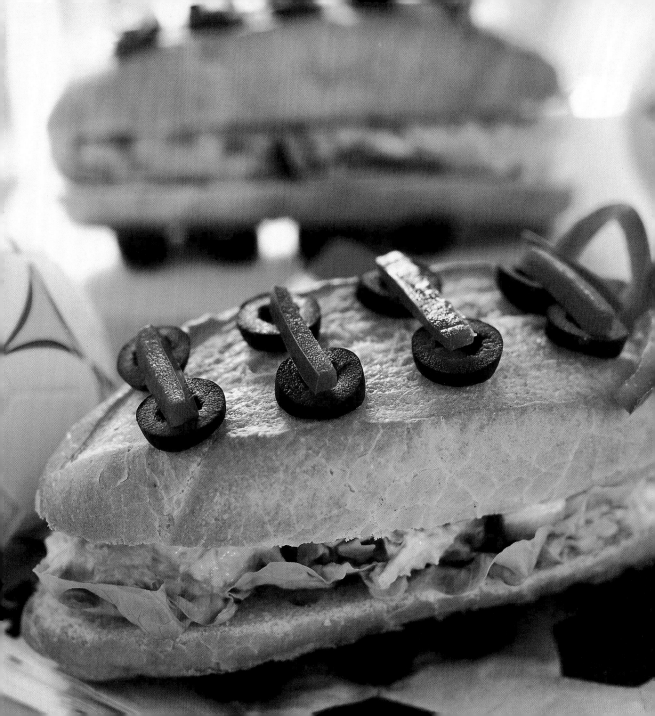

Soccer Shoe Baguettes

These would be great to serve as a snack when a big soccer game is on and would be perfect for a soccer party. I have chosen a tuna salad filling, but there are many other choices like cheese and tomato, turkey salad, and ham and cheese.

To make the filling, drain and flake the tuna and mix it together with the celery and mayonnaise. Cut the baguettes in half lengthwise and spread with butter. Line with lettuce leaves and spoon some of the filling on top. Arrange some sliced tomatoes and cucumber on top.

PLACE THE BAGUETTES on halved black olives to represent the cleats of the soccer shoes. Thinly slice some of the olives to use as eyelets and place on top of the baguettes. Use thin slices as well as circles of bell pepper to represent laces.

MAKES 4 MINI BAGUETTES

Two 6-ounce cans tuna
  in oil

1 celery stalk, finely chopped

2 to 3 tablespoons
  mayonnaise

4 small baguettes or 2 large
  baguettes cut in half

Butter

Lettuce

Tomato slices

Cucumber slices

Black olives, pitted

1 red bell pepper

Mini Baked Potatoes

Prick small red or white potatoes (not baking potatoes) with a fork. Brush with oil and sprinkle with salt. Bake in an oven preheated to 400°F for 45 to 55 minutes until crisp on the outside and tender inside.

SERVES 6

COCKTAIL SAUCE
1 tablespoon ketchup
1½ tablespoons mayonnaise
½ teaspoon Worcestershire
  sauce
Few drops of Tabasco sauce
Pinch of celery salt (optional)
1 tablespoon heavy cream
Salt and white pepper

1 large avocado, peeled,
  pitted, and diced
½ pound fresh cooked shrimp
Cucumber slices

There are many simple toppings for baked potatoes, such as grated cheese and ham, sour cream and chives, and broccoli and Cheddar. However, for something a little different, try the three ideas given here.

Avocado and Shrimp Cocktail Topping

Mix together all the ingredients to make the cocktail sauce. Combine the avocado and shrimp and mix thoroughly with the sauce. Cut crosses in the tops of the baked potatoes, spoon in the topping, and decorate with a cucumber slice on a toothpick to form a sail.

Mexican Chicken Topping

You could use Old El Paso fajita seasoning mix instead of the oregano and chili powder.

Mix the chicken with the chili powder, oregano, 1½ teaspoons of the olive oil, and some salt and pepper. Heat the remaining 1½ teaspoons oil in a pan and sauté the onion for 1 minute or until beginning to soften. Add the chicken and sauté for about 4 minutes until cooked through. Stir in the tomato. Cut crosses in the tops of the baked potatoes, spoon in the topping, top with sour cream and salsa, and decorate each one with a tortilla chip sail.

SERVES 4

1 boneless, skinless chicken breast, finely diced

Generous pinch of mild chili powder

¼ teaspoon dried oregano

1 tablespoon olive oil

Salt and freshly ground black pepper

½ small onion, chopped

1 ripe tomato, diced

2 tablespoons sour cream

2 tablespoons salsa

Tortilla chips

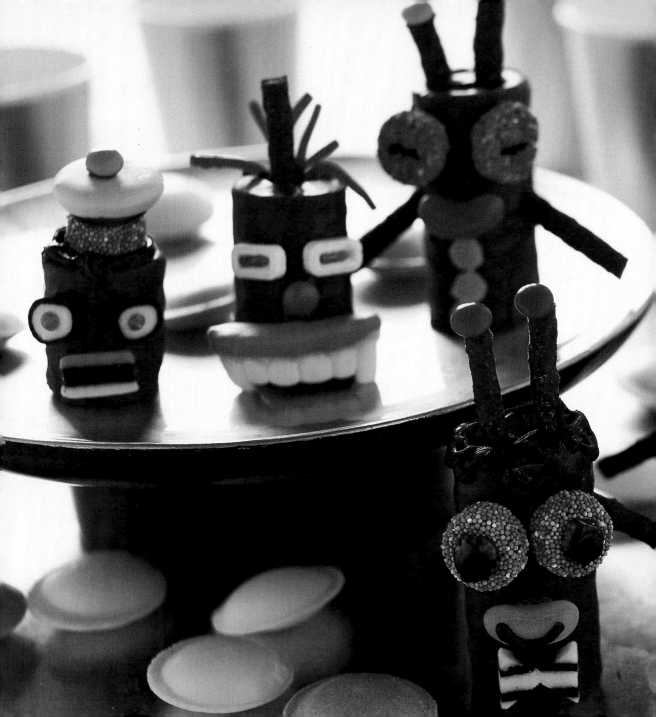

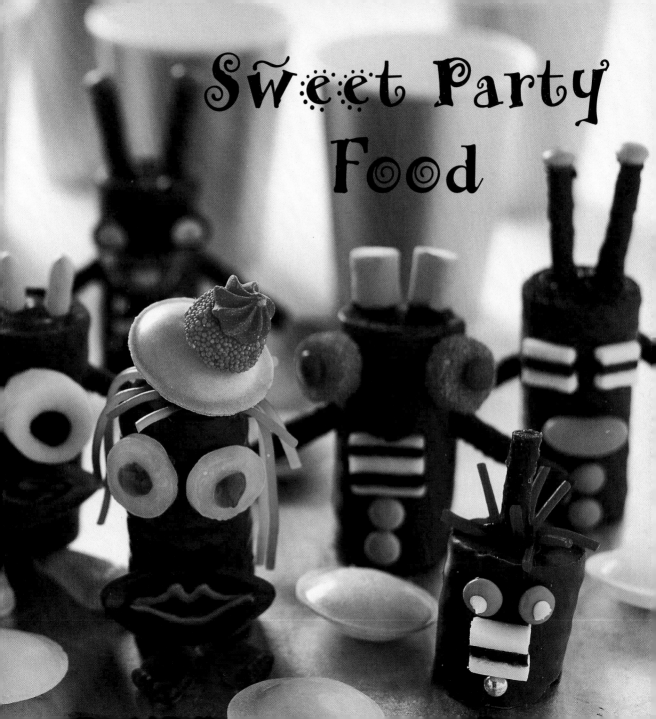

Sweet Party Food

Chocolate Aliens

MAKES AS MANY AS YOU LIKE

Ho Hos or Yodels

Tubes of colored writing icing

Variety of candies

Create your very own edible extraterrestrials.

Decorate the Ho Hos or Yodels as in the photograph on the previous pages to look like aliens, using writing icing and a variety of candies attached with melted chocolate.

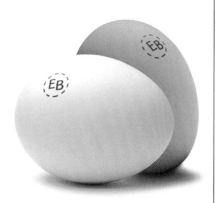

When using eggs, choose Eggland's Best; they contain ten times the vitamin E of ordinary eggs, 25 percent less saturated fat, and 100 milligrams of omega-3, three times more than ordinary eggs. They are also lower in cholesterol. EB eggs come from hens fed a patented, all-natural, all-vegetarian diet with no animal fats, no animal by-products, no steroids, and no added hormones or antibiotics of any kind. The feed contains only healthy grains, canola oil, and an all-natural supplement of rice bran, kelp, alfalfa, and vitamin E. The EB stamped on the shells is your assurance that the eggs meet the high standards of taste, nutrition, and quality established for EB. A healthier lifestyle awaits you and your family if you use Eggland's Best eggs.

Try these egg experiments with your children.

How do you know your eggs are fresh?
Place the egg in a glass or a small bowl of water. If it stays at the bottom it is very fresh. If it tilts up slightly it is up to a week old. If it floats, throw it away.

How can you tell if an egg is hard-boiled?
Spin the egg on a flat surface. Place your finger on top of the egg to stop it moving and then take it away immediately. If the egg is raw it continues to spin.

OVERLEAF: Chocolate Aliens

My Favorite Chocolate Cake

This is the most delicious chocolate cake—moist and lovely and chocolaty. It is also very easy and quick to make.

Preheat the oven to 350°F. Cream together the butter or margarine and sugar until light and fluffy. Beat the eggs and mix with the cocoa powder. Gradually add the egg and cocoa powder mixture to the creamed butter and sugar. Sift together the flour and baking powder and fold this into the batter, then gradually mix in the milk until well blended. Line with waxed paper and grease two 8-inch round baking pans and spoon the mixture into each of them. Bake for about 30 minutes until risen and slightly firm to the touch. Allow to cool a little, remove from the pans, and place on a wire cooling rack.

TO PREPARE THE FUDGE TOPPING, heat the cream in a saucepan until boiling. Remove from the heat and stir in the broken chocolate until melted. Finally, beat in the butter. Allow to cool and place in the fridge for about 30 minutes before using to sandwich the cakes together and also to cover the top and sides of the cake. Decorate with piped rosettes of cream, fresh raspberries, and mint.

SERVES 8

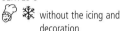 without the icing and decoration

1 stick unsalted butter or
½ cup soft margarine

2 cups light brown sugar

2 large eggs

½ cup Dutch-process cocoa
powder

1⅔ cups self-rising flour

1 teaspoon baking powder

1 cup milk

FUDGE TOPPING

¾ cup heavy cream

8 ounces bittersweet
chocolate, broken into pieces

2 tablespoons unsalted butter,
diced

DECORATION

¾ cup heavy cream, whipped

Fresh raspberries

Fresh mint leaves

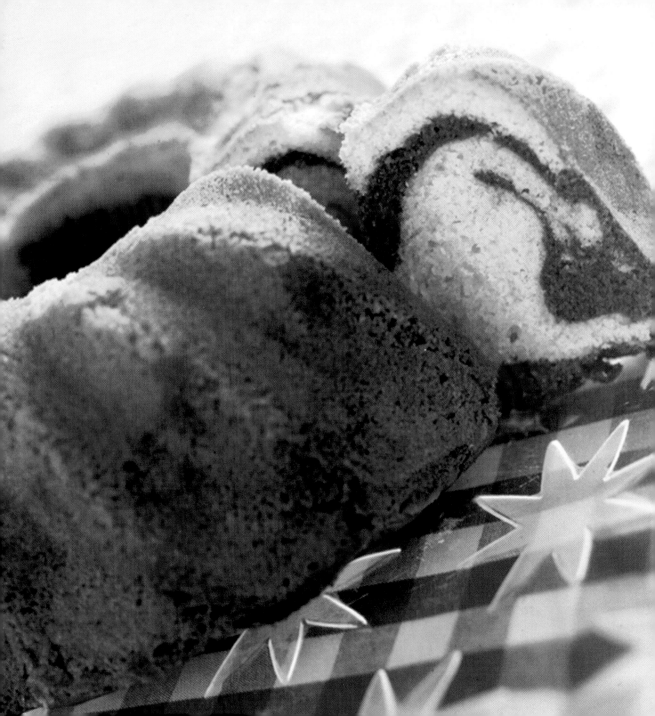

Nicholas's Favorite Marble Cake

My son, Nicholas, likes to help me make this cake and really enjoys the bit where you swirl the colors together, but I have to temper his enthusiasm or the whole cake can turn a murky brown.

Preheat the oven to 325°F. Cream the butter and sugar together until fluffy. Sift together the almonds and flour and add to the mixture. Gradually beat in the eggs, one at a time, and add the milk. Transfer half the cake mixture to another bowl and stir in the almond extract and orange zest. Melt the chocolate in a microwave or double boiler, and stir the melted chocolate and cocoa powder into the remaining cake mixture.

THIS CAKE LOOKS BEST when baked in a fluted 8-inch-diameter Bundt pan. Grease and flour the pan first or use a nonstick baking spray. Alternatively, line a loaf pan or an 8-inch round pan with parchment or other baking paper and pour in the batter. Spoon alternate layers of the cake batters into the pan and use a skewer or a knife to swirl through the mixture to give a marbled effect. Level the surface and bake for about 1 hour until the cake is well risen and golden. Turn out onto a wire rack and let cool.

SERVES 10

❄ **N**

2 sticks unsalted butter, at room temperature

1 cup plus 2 tablespoons superfine sugar

1 cup ground almonds

1 cup plus 2 tablespoons self-rising flour, sifted

4 large eggs

3 tablespoons milk

1 teaspoon almond extract

1 teaspoon finely grated orange zest

3 ounces bittersweet chocolate, broken into small pieces, or bittersweet chocolate chips

1 tablespoon Dutch-process cocoa powder, sifted

Heart-Shaped Faces

MAKES 18 COOKIES

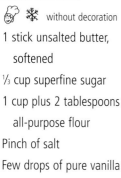 without decoration

1 stick unsalted butter,
   softened
⅓ cup superfine sugar
1 cup plus 2 tablespoons
   all-purpose flour
Pinch of salt
Few drops of pure vanilla
   extract

GLACÉ ICING
1½ cups confectioners' sugar,
   sifted
About 1½ tablespoons lemon
   juice or water

DECORATION
Assorted tubes of writing icing
Mini colored sugar balls

It's fun to make and decorate these to look like different members of the family and friends for Mother's Day.

Preheat the oven to 350°F. Beat the butter and sugar together either by hand with a wooden spoon or in an electric mixer at low speed until thoroughly mixed. Sift together the flour and salt and mix into the butter mixture together with the vanilla to form a fairly stiff dough. If the dough is too dry, add a little water.

Form the dough into a ball and then roll out thinly on a floured work surface using a rolling pin dusted with flour. Cut into heart shapes using cookie cutters. Collect all the trimmings together and roll these out again to make more cookies. Arrange on greased or waxed-paper-lined baking sheets and bake for about 15 minutes until the cookies are lightly golden.

TO MAKE THE GLACÉ ICING, put the confectioners' sugar in a bowl and add enough lemon juice or water to make a good spreading consistency. Spread the icing onto the cooled cookies with a spatula or small blunt knife. When they are set, decorate each cookie to look like a face.

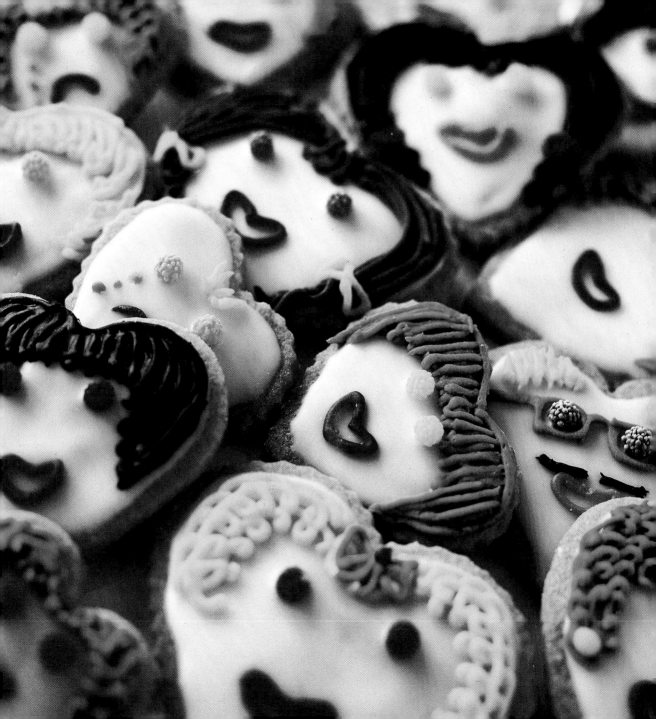

Carrot and Pineapple Muffins

MAKES 12 REGULAR OR ABOUT 30

MINI MUFFINS

¾ cup all-purpose flour

¾ cup whole-wheat flour

1 teaspoon baking powder

¾ teaspoon baking soda

1½ teaspoons ground
   cinnamon

½ teaspoon salt

¾ cup plus 2 tablespoons
   canola oil

½ cup superfine sugar

2 large eggs

¾ cup finely grated carrot

1 cup canned crushed
   pineapple, drained but with
   some juice

¾ cup raisins

These are probably my favorite muffins; they are wonderfully moist with an irresistible taste. They make a good snack any time of the day and also make great mini muffins for parties. It is a good idea to cut the raisins in half when making mini muffins.

Preheat the oven to 350°F. Sift together the flours, baking powder, baking soda, cinnamon, and salt and mix well. Beat the oil, sugar, and eggs in a separate bowl until well blended. Add the grated carrot, crushed pineapple, and raisins. Gradually add the flour mixture, beating until the ingredients are just combined.

POUR THE BATTER INTO 12 MUFFIN CUPS lined with paper liners and bake for 25 minutes for regular muffins (15 to 17 minutes for mini muffins). Allow to cool for a few minutes, then remove the muffins from the cups in their liners and let cool on a wire rack.

Coconut Kisses

I defy you to eat only one of these! They are definitely one of my favorites, and your children will enjoy helping you make them as well as eat them.

Preheat the oven to 350°F. Cream together the butter and sugars. Add the egg and vanilla. Sift together the flour, baking soda, and salt and beat this into the mixture. Stir in the chocolate chips, oats, and coconut.

FORM INTO WALNUT-SIZE BALLS, flatten the tops with your hand, and place 2½ inches apart on a lightly greased or lined baking pans. Bake for 14 to 15 minutes. The cookies will harden when they cool down.

MAKES 25 COOKIES

1 stick unsalted butter

⅓ cup light brown sugar

⅓ cup superfine sugar

1 large egg, lightly beaten

½ teaspoon pure vanilla extract

½ cup plus 2 tablespoons all-purpose flour

½ teaspoon baking soda

½ teaspoon salt

¾ cup bittersweet chocolate chips

1 cup rolled oats

½ cup sweetened flaked coconut

Annabel's Apricot Cookies

MAKES 26 COOKIES

1 stick unsalted butter

4 ounces cream cheese

½ cup superfine sugar

¾ cup all-purpose flour

½ cup chopped dried apricots

½ cup white chocolate chips
  or chopped white chocolate

This fabulous and rather unusual combination of dried apricots and white chocolate makes irresistible cookies. Once you have sampled these, you will probably want to double the quantities the second time around.

Preheat the oven to 350°F. In a large mixing bowl, cream together the butter and cream cheese. Add the sugar and beat until fluffy. Gradually add the flour, then fold in the apricots and chocolate. The dough will be quite soft—don't worry!

DROP THE MIXTURE BY HEAPING teaspoons onto baking sheets and bake for 15 minutes or until lightly golden. Allow the cookies to cool and harden for a few minutes before removing from the baking sheet.

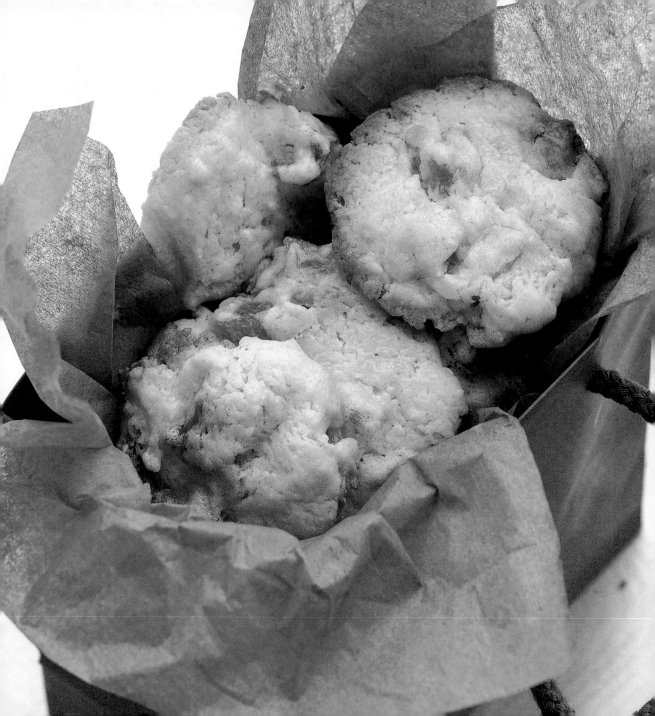

Apple Smiles

MAKES 4 APPLE SMILES

 N

Creamy peanut butter

1 red apple, cored and sliced
   into eighths

Squeeze of lemon juice

Miniature marshmallows or
   small cubes of cheese (for a
   healthier alternative)

Dried apricots (optional)

This snack is easy to prepare and will certainly bring a smile to your child's face! For a healthier variation, use small cubes of banana instead of mini marshmallows.

Spread peanut butter on one side of each apple slice (squeeze a little lemon juice over the apple slices first if not serving immediately). Place five marshmallows or cubes of cheese on one apple slice and lay another apple slice, peanut butter side down, on top. If you like, add an apricot to form the tongue.

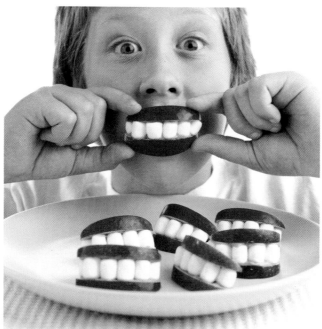

S'mores

These no-bake chocolate, fruit, nut, and marshmallow treats are amazingly good, and they are also fun for children to make themselves.

Put the chocolate and butter into a large heatproof bowl and place over a pan of simmering water; stir occasionally until melted. Stir the condensed milk into the chocolate mixture and mix in the graham crackers, raisins, apricots, ½ cup of the mini marshmallows, and the chopped pecans

To MAKE THE BARS, line a 9 x 13-inch shallow cake pan with plastic wrap, allowing the sides to overhang. Spoon the mixture into the pan and press down but still leave the top a little rough. Scatter the remaining ¼ cup marshmallows over the top. Place in the fridge for about an hour to set. Once set, lift the cake out of the pan by the overhanging plastic wrap and cut into bars. Keep chilled in the fridge.

MAKES 12 BARS

 N

8 ounces bittersweet
    chocolate, broken
    into pieces
6 tablespoons unsalted butter,
    cut into pieces
One 14-ounce can
    condensed milk
8 ounces graham crackers
    (about 20), broken into
    small pieces
⅓ cup raisins
⅓ cup chopped dried apricots
¾ cup mini marshmallows
¼ cup chopped pecans

Glossy Dark and White Chocolate Brownies

MAKES 16 SQUARES

5 ounces dark chocolate
  (semisweet or bittersweet),
  chopped

6 tablespoons unsalted butter

1 teaspoon pure vanilla extract

½ cup superfine sugar

2 large eggs

1 large egg yolk

⅔ cup all-purpose flour

¼ teaspoon salt

1 cup white chocolate chips

CHOCOLATE SATIN GLAZE

3 ounces bittersweet
  chocolate, chopped

1 tablespoon unsalted butter

½ cup white chocolate chips

Two chocolates are combined to make these irresistible squares of rich, chewy brownies.

Preheat the oven to 350°F, and line with waxed paper and grease an 8-inch square baking pan. Put the dark chocolate and butter in a bowl and microwave for 2 minutes on high (or melt in a saucepan over low heat, stirring constantly). Stir in the vanilla and sugar, then add the eggs and yolk, one at a time, stirring after each addition. Sift together the flour and salt and mix this into the chocolate mixture with the white chocolate chips. Pour the batter into the prepared pan and bake for about 30 minutes.

To PREPARE THE GLAZE, melt the dark chocolate and butter together in a small heatproof bowl over a pan of simmering water and spread over the brownies. Melt the white chocolate chips in a bowl over a pan of simmering water and, using a teaspoon, trail five lines horizontally across the cake about ½ inch apart. Alternatively, pipe lines of white chocolate. Then, with a blunt knife, draw vertical lines lightly through the chocolate glaze to create a pattern. Cut into 16 squares.

Yummy Gelatin Boats

These gelatin boats are probably the most popular party food that I make.

Squeeze the juice from the oranges and reserve for fresh juice to drink. Carefully scrape out the membrane and discard, taking care not to make a hole in the skin of the orange. Prepare the gelatin according to the package instructions, but use ¾ cup boiling water instead of 1 cup, and fill each of the hollow orange halves with gelatin right to the top. Refrigerate until set and then cut the oranges in half again with a sharp wet knife. Cut triangles out of the rice paper and secure with toothpicks to make sails.

MAKES 8 BOATS

2 large oranges, halved
One 3-ounce package gelatin
   dessert, strawberry, orange,
   or lime
2 sheets rice paper
8 toothpicks

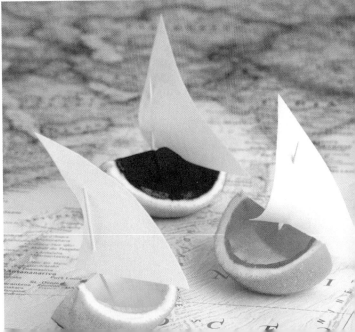

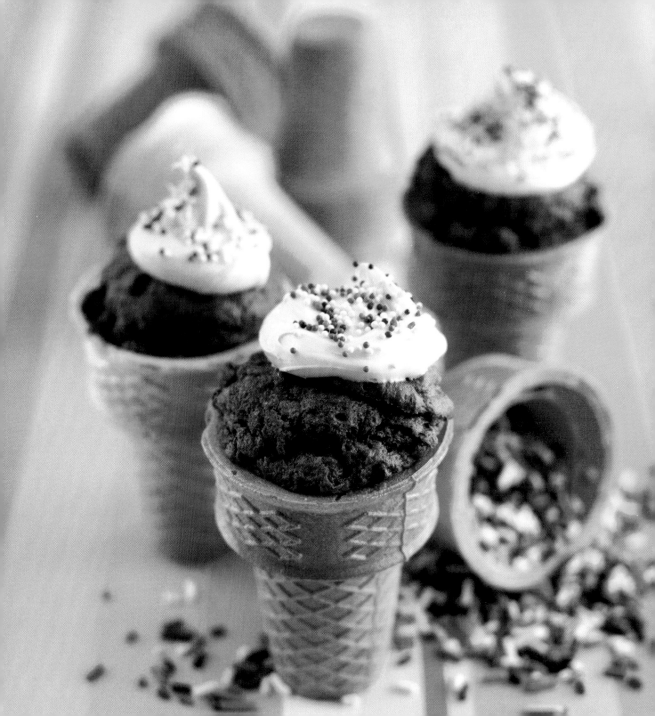

Chocolate Muffin Ice-Cream Cones

A fun way to present chocolate muffins is to bake them in flat-bottomed ice-cream cones, which you can buy in the supermarket. You can cheat by using a package of muffin mix.

Add the cocoa powder to the muffin mix. Following the package instructions, mix together the water, oil, and eggs and stir in the muffin mix.

PREHEAT THE OVEN TO 350°F. Wrap foil around the cone bases and place upright in an ungreased muffin pan. Fill each cone with about 3 tablespoons of the muffin mixture. Do not overfill the cone or it may bake over the sides. Gently tap the bottoms of the cones with your hand to settle the batter.

PLACE THE CONES IN THE OVEN and bake for about 20 minutes. Allow to cool completely. Ice the tops with vanilla frosting that you have tinted with assorted food coloring, and decorate with colored sprinkles.

MAKES 12 CONES

2 tablespoons Dutch-process cocoa powder

One 18.25-ounce package Betty Crocker Double Chocolate Muffin Mix

¾ cup water

¼ cup canola oil

2 large eggs

12 flat-bottomed ice-cream cones without holes or cracks

One 16-ounce tub vanilla frosting (Betty Crocker Rich & Creamy Frosting)

Assorted food coloring

Colored sprinkles for decoration

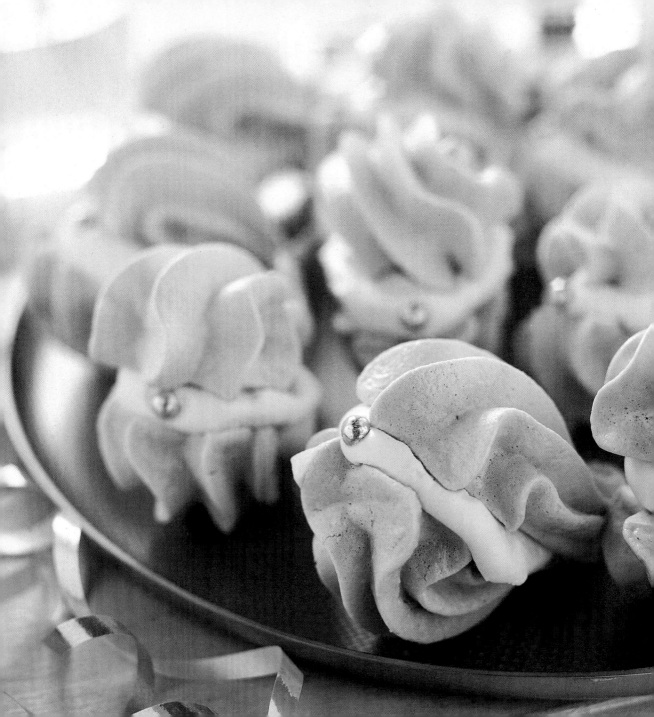

Pink Meringue Shells

These look like oyster shells with pearls inside. Present them on a plate with a Little Mermaid doll in the center.

MAKES 20 PAIRS OF MERINGUE SHELLS

3 large egg whites
¾ cup superfine sugar
Few drops of pink food coloring
1 cup heavy cream
Edible silver balls, or pink jelly beans

Preheat the oven to 225°F. Whisk the egg whites until firm. Continue to whisk while adding 1 tablespoon of the sugar at a time and using up half the sugar. Using a wooden spoon, fold in the remaining sugar together with the food coloring. Spoon the mixture into a pastry bag fitted with a ½-inch star tip. Pipe about 40 small shell shapes onto baking pans lined with parchment or other nonstick baking paper. Bake the meringues for about 1 hour 40 minutes until crisp. Arrange the meringues on a wire rack to cool.

TO CREATE THE FINISHED EFFECT, whip the cream until it forms stiff peaks and use it to sandwich together pairs of meringue shells. Place a silver ball, a "pearl," in the middle of each open shell.

Tip

Egg whites will whisk better for meringue if they are at room temperature, so take them out of the fridge an hour or so before use.

Makeup and Jewelry Party

This party will indulge every little girl's fantasy—after all, if your daughters are anything like my two girls, they can't wait to see what they would look like wearing makeup, high heels, and Mommy's costume jewelry.

Decide on how many children you want to invite—you will probably want to make this an all-girls' party. You can ask them on the invitation to wear their most trendy outfits.

Start collecting inexpensive makeup like glittery nail polish, nail polish remover, eye shadow, mascara, and lipstick, and makeup brushes, hair ornaments, spray-on hair color, etc. Also ask your friends if they have any makeup they don't want anymore. Have some towels to drape around the children's shoulders to protect their clothes as they are made up.

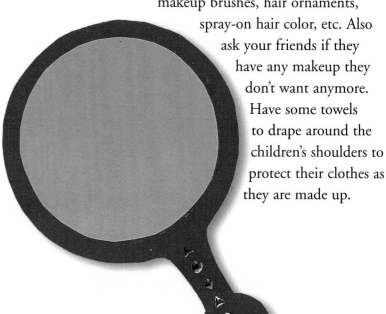

You will need some helpers—teenage girls would be great to assist you in the beauty salon. Put a big mirror in front of the children so that they can see what is going on.

Organize different areas for makeup, hair, and nail polish. While the girls are waiting their turns, have a collection of beads and thread for them to make necklaces and bracelets to wear.

Once everyone has been made up, serve snacks, and afterward you could organize party games. It is a good idea to take "before" and "after" photographs of each of the children. You could make a little booth in a corner of a room with a chair and a sign behind it saying SCARLETT'S BEAUTY SALON. Print the photographs and send them out with your daughter's thank-you cards.

Adding to the Fun

Have an appointment book where the children reserve who they want to do their makeup, hair, and nails and give them a number so that they know when it is their turn.

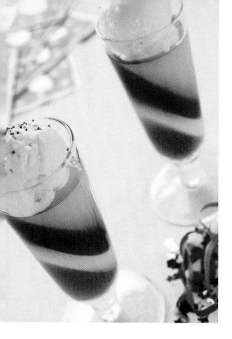

Tilted Gelatins

These look fantastic and everyone will want to know how you got the gelatin to set in diagonal stripes. If you like, add some fruit such as canned mandarin oranges or fresh raspberries to the various gelatins, but when it comes to green, don't use kiwi, as it contains something that prevents gelatin from setting.

MAKES 4 TALL GLASSES

Four 3-ounce packages
   assorted gelatin desserts,
   such as strawberry, lime,
   black cherry, and orange
4 scoops ice cream
Colored sprinkles

Prepare half of each package of gelatin in separate bowls according to the package instructions. Divide the strawberry gelatin among four tall glasses and then chill the glasses in the fridge set at an angle. Repeat with the next two gelatins, each time propping the glasses at an angle so that the gelatin sets on a diagonal, and allow setting time between each. Pour in the last gelatin, and this time stand the glass upright. When the last gelatin has set, add a scoop of ice cream and decorate with sprinkles.

Goldfish Bowl Gelatin

If you really want to make this look like the real thing, you could always put a few drops of blue food coloring into the gelatin.

Prepare one package of gelatin according to the instructions on the package. Pour it into a round glass bowl that looks like a goldfish bowl. Set aside in the fridge until thickened and then push in about six gummy fish so that they look as though they are swimming around in the bowl. Place in the fridge until almost set. Prepare the second package of gelatin, pour into the bowl, and then return to the fridge until completely set.

MAKES 1 GOLDFISH BOWL

Two 3-ounce packages yellow
or green gelatin dessert
Gummy fish

OVERLEAF: Chocolate Profiterole Cats (page 86), Goldfish Bowl Gelatin (this page)

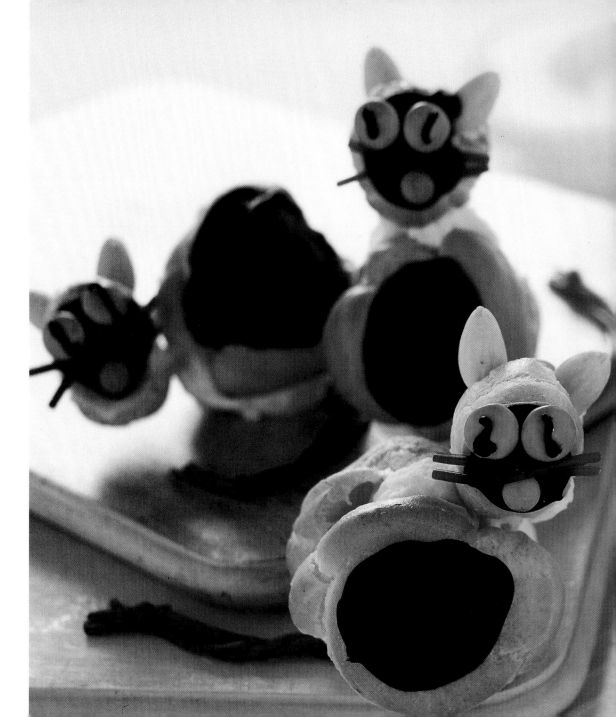

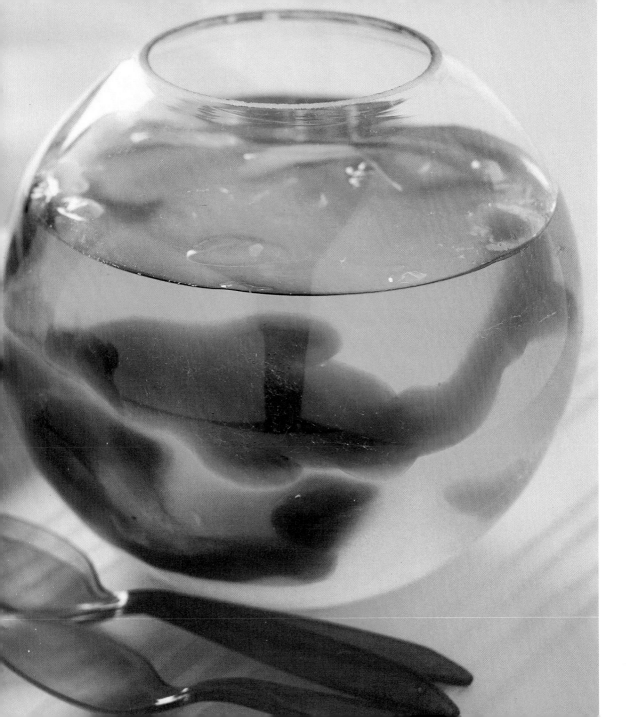

Chocolate Profiterole Cats

MAKES 11 LARGE AND 11 SMALL
PROFITEROLES OR 11 CAT
PROFITEROLES

❄ without the chocolate **N**

6 tablespoons unsalted butter

1 cup water

¾ cup all-purpose flour

¼ cup superfine sugar

Pinch of salt

3 large eggs, lightly beaten

1 pint good-quality ice cream

4½ to 5 ounces dark or milk
    chocolate

DECORATION

1 tube black writing icing

Mini M&M's

Whole almonds

Licorice laces

It's not difficult to make choux pastry for profiteroles. By fitting a plain round nozzle into a pastry bag, you can also pipe the pastry into mini éclairs and fill with ice cream. For a real novelty, make large and small rounds of pastry and stack these on top of each other to look like pussy cats. These cats can be made ahead and frozen, and then all you will need to do is add the finishing touches to the decoration.

To make the choux pastry, preheat the oven to 400°F. Put the butter and water in a saucepan and slowly bring to a boil. Sift the flour onto waxed or parchment or other baking paper—this will enable you to slide it in all at once, which is important for making a smooth mixture. Add the flour, sugar, and salt and then beat vigorously with a wooden spoon until the mixture comes away from the sides of the saucepan. Allow to cool slightly and beat in half the eggs. Gradually beat in the remainder of the eggs (you may not need to use all of the eggs) to make a glossy smooth dough that has a thick dropping consistency.

Grease and flour two large baking sheets. Drop 11 tablespoonfuls and 11 smaller spoonfuls of the mixture onto the sheets. (They will increase in size quite a bit once they are baked.) Bake for 25 minutes or until risen and golden. Pierce each cream puff with a skewer or the point of a sharp knife to release the steam, then return to the oven for 5 to 10 minutes to crisp. Allow the puffs to cool on a wire rack.

When cool, cut a slit in the puffs and fill with ice cream. Pop them in the freezer while you melt the chocolate over a pan of simmering water. Dip each of the puffs in the melted chocolate to coat the top.

TO MAKE CAT PROFITEROLES, attach a small puff on top of a larger puff with a little of the melted chocolate. With the black writing icing, draw a line down the center of green M&M's and stick these on the face for eyes and use pink M&M's for the nose. Make two little slits in the top of the small puff and stick in almonds for the ears. Finish off by attaching a strip of licorice for each cat's whiskers and tail. Store in the freezer and allow to defrost a little before eating.

Jam Tarts

MAKES ABOUT 24 JAM TARTS

1½ cups all-purpose flour

Pinch of salt

1 stick unsalted butter, diced

½ cup confectioners' sugar

1 large egg, lightly beaten

Strawberry, raspberry, cherry,
   or other jam of your choice

These have always been a real favorite with children. Nothing tastes quite as good as the homemade version.

Sift the flour and salt together. Rub in the butter with your fingertips until the mixture resembles fine bread crumbs. Mix in the sugar. Stir in the egg until the mixture forms a soft dough. Form into a ball using your hands and wrap in plastic wrap. Set aside in the fridge for about 30 minutes; this prevents the pastry from shrinking when it is baked.

TO MAKE THE TARTS, roll out the dough on a lightly floured surface and cut into about 24 circles using a 3½-inch round fluted cutter. Lightly grease two muffin pans and press in the dough circles. Put back in the fridge for about 20 minutes. Preheat the oven to 400°F. Fill each tart with about 2 teaspoons jam and bake for about 15 minutes.

Buzzy Bees

These bees, packed full of tasty ingredients, are great fun for parties. They are just the right size for little children. Older children will enjoy making these themselves because they are quick and easy to assemble and need no cooking. You may want to double the quantity next time, since these bees will keep your children buzzing around for more.

MAKES 10 BEES

N

¼ cup creamy peanut butter

1 tablespoon honey

2 tablespoons nonfat dry milk

1 tablespoon sesame seeds

1 shredded wheat biscuit, crushed

DECORATION

1 tablespoon cocoa powder

Sliced almonds, or rice paper cut into the shape of wings

10 raisins or currants

Mix together the peanut butter and honey, then blend in the remaining ingredients. Form heaping teaspoons of the mixture into oval shapes to look like bees. To decorate, dip a toothpick into the cocoa powder and press gently onto the bees' bodies to form stripes. Press sliced almonds or rice paper wings into the sides of the bees. Cut the raisins or currants in half, roll between your finger and thumb to form tiny balls, and arrange them on the bees to look like eyes. The bees can be stored in the fridge for several days.

White Chocolate Rice Krispies Squares

MAKES 12 SQUARES

6 tablespoons unsalted butter

¼ cup corn syrup or golden syrup, such as Lyle's

½ cup white chocolate chips

3 cups Rice Krispies

½ cup pastel-colored mini marshmallows

For those with less than ten minutes to spare, here is a great recipe that is adored by my three children.

Put the butter, corn or golden syrup, and white chocolate into a small saucepan and melt together over low heat. Transfer to a bowl and set aside to cool. Mix together the Rice Krispies and marshmallows and stir in the syrup mixture. Line a fairly shallow 8-inch square baking pan with waxed paper, spoon in the mixture, and level the surface. Cut into squares and store in the fridge.

Rice Krispies Squares

MAKES 16 SQUARES

Three 2-ounce Milky Way bars

6 tablespoons unsalted butter

2½ cups Rice Krispies

⅓ cup raisins

Here is a fine and tasty variation on the theme.

Cut the candy bars into pieces, put into a saucepan with the butter, and melt over low heat. In a bowl, combine the Rice Krispies and raisins. Stir the melted Milky Way bars into the Rice Krispies until well coated. Press into an 8-inch square pan, and finish as above.

Chocolate and Toffee Rice Krispies Squares

Here is a truly scrumptious recipe for your children to share among their friends.

Line the base of an 8-inch square pan with waxed paper and grease the sides. Put the syrup, sugar, and butter in a saucepan and stir over low heat until melted. Remove from the heat and stir in the Rice Krispies. Press this mixture into the prepared pan.

TO MAKE THE FILLING, put the toffees, butter, and cream into a saucepan. Stir over low heat until melted. Bring to a boil and pour on top of the Rice Krispies mixture. Put in the fridge to set for about 1 hour.

FOR THE TOPPING, break the chocolate into pieces and put it into a heatproof bowl together with the butter. Place over a pan of simmering water and stir until melted. Alternatively, melt the chocolate and butter in a suitable dish in the microwave. Spread the topping over the toffee filling and set aside in the fridge for about 1 hour until set. Carefully remove from the pan, peel off the paper, and cut into squares. Store in the fridge.

MAKES 16 SQUARES

¼ cup corn syrup or golden
   syrup, such as Lyle's
⅓ packed cup light brown
   sugar
3 tablespoons unsalted butter
2 cups Rice Krispies

TOFFEE FILLING

1 cup toffee candies
4 tablespoons unsalted butter
3 tablespoons heavy cream

TOPPING

3 ounces dark or milk
   chocolate
2 tablespoons unsalted butter

This Little Piggy Went to the Party

SERVES 10

1 round watermelon
1 cantaloupe
1 honeydew melon
Red and green grapes

DECORATION
2 large limes
Toothpicks
2 glacé (candied) cherries
2 raisins

This is such an amazing way to serve fruit and is always greeted with squeals of delight!

Mark with a pencil or pen the spiral tail of the pig on the watermelon. Cut around the tail and then cut out a large round hole from the top of the melon. Remove the cutout sections and use them to cut a 2-inch-diameter circle for the snout of the pig and two triangles for the ears. Stick two melon seeds into the center of the snout for the nostrils and set aside.

Using a melon baller, scoop out the watermelon until the shell is empty. Discard the seeds as you go. Scrape out any remaining melon and drain any juice. Mop up any remaining juice inside the shell with paper towels. Cut the other two melons in half, remove the seeds, and scoop out melon balls. Add to the watermelon balls in a large bowl. Add the grapes.

TO DECORATE THE WATERMELON, halve the limes and attach with toothpicks for the feet. Attach the snout and ears with toothpicks. Slice the ends off the cherries, push a raisin into the center of each, and attach with toothpicks to form the eyes. Drain any liquid from the fruits and fill the watermelon shell.

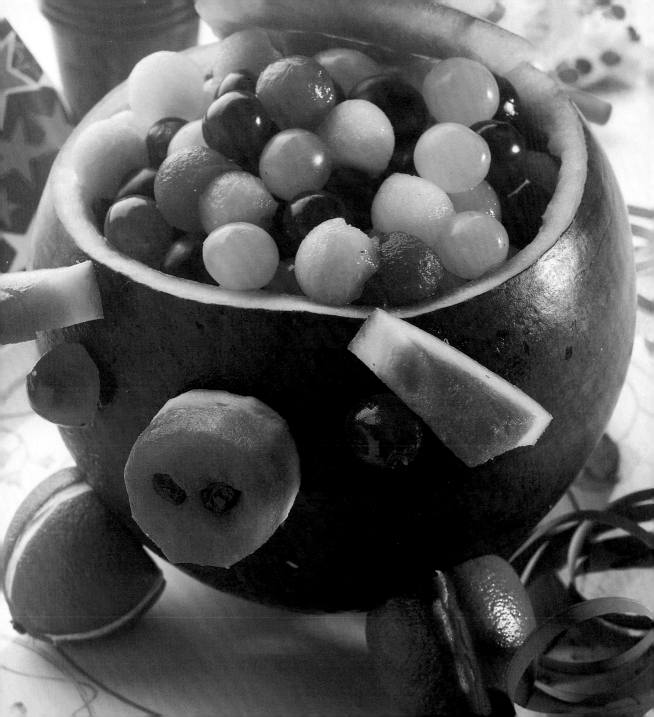

White Chocolate-Chunk Cookies

MAKES 20 COOKIES

 N ❄

1 stick unsalted butter

1 cup confectioners' sugar

½ cup light brown sugar

1 large egg

1 teaspoon pure vanilla extract

1 cup plus 2 tablespoons
   all-purpose flour

½ teaspoon baking powder

¼ teaspoon salt

6 ounces white chocolate,
   broken into small chunks

⅔ cup finely chopped pecans
   or walnuts (optional)

These are very easy to make and one of my favorite cookies. They should be quite soft when they are taken out of the oven so that when they cool down, they are crisp on the outside but moist and chewy inside. Leave out the nuts for young children.

Preheat the oven to 375°F. Beat the butter together with the sugars. With a fork, beat the egg together with the vanilla and add to the butter mixture. In a bowl, mix together the flour, baking powder, and salt. Add to the butter and egg mixture and blend well. Mix in the chunks of white chocolate and the nuts, if using.

To make the cookies, line several baking sheets with parchment or other nonstick baking paper. Using your hands, form the dough into walnut-size balls and arrange on the baking sheets, spaced well apart. Bake for 10 to 12 minutes. Allow to cool for a few minutes and then transfer to wire racks.

Blondies

These are called blondies and not brownies because they are made with white chocolate. Blondies always crack a little on the surface, so, if you like, you can sift some confectioners' sugar over the surface. To cut the blondies into neat squares, put the whole cake on a board when it has cooled completely and cut into nine large or sixteen smaller squares. The blondies will keep for up to a week in an airtight container.

Preheat the oven to 375°F, and grease and line with parchment or other baking paper an 8-inch square baking pan. Melt 4 ounces of the white chocolate with the butter in a heatproof bowl over a pan of simmering water. Set aside to cool down. Beat the eggs with the sugar until smooth, then gradually beat in the melted chocolate mixture. Sift together the flour and salt, then fold into the egg mixture together with the remaining white chocolate, the pecans, and the vanilla.

MAKE THE BLONDIES by spooning the mixture into the prepared pan; level the surface with a spatula. Bake for 30 to 35 minutes until risen and golden and the center is just firm to the touch. Leave to cool in the pan, then turn out onto a wire rack. When completely cool, cut into squares.

MAKES 9 LARGE OR 16 SMALL
  BLONDIES

N

10 ounces white chocolate,
  chopped

6 tablespoons unsalted butter,
  diced

3 large eggs

¾ cup superfine sugar

1 cup plus 2 tablesoons
  self-rising flour

Pinch of salt

1 cup chopped pecans

1 teaspoon pure vanilla extract

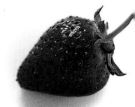

Party Drinks

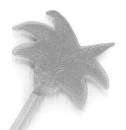

Serve any of these drinks with orange or pineapple slices and maraschino cherries on toothpicks, paper umbrellas, and fancy straws. These drinks are fun for children to mix up themselves.

Exotic Fruit Cocktail

MAKES 2 GLASSES
1 cup lemonade
½ cup mixed tropical fruit juice
2 tablespoons grenadine or
   strawberry syrup
2 pineapple wedges
2 maraschino cherries

This looks good because the colors of the drink separate due to the different densities of the liquids. You could make pink lemonade by mixing lemonade with a little of the grenadine syrup.

Pour the lemonade into two glasses, pour the fruit juice down the sides of each glass, then pour a tablespoon of the syrup down the sides. Decorate with a wedge of pineapple and a cherry on a toothpick and add a straw.

Strawberry Milkshake

MAKES 2 GLASSES
A handful of strawberries
4 scoops strawberry ice cream
1 tablespoon strawberry syrup
1 cup milk

Puree the strawberries and strain. Combine the strawberry puree with 2 scoops of softened ice cream, the syrup, and milk. Pour into two glasses and add a scoop of ice cream to each. Place an umbrella in the ice cream and add a straw.

Ice Cream Soda

Blend together the fruit cocktail, soda, and two scoops of the vanilla ice cream. Pour into two tall glasses, place a scoop of ice cream on top of each, and add a straw and the orange and cherry on a toothpick for decoration.

MAKES 2 GLASSES

One 4-ounce cup fruit cocktail, drained

1 cup Sprite or 7UP

4 scoops vanilla ice cream

2 slices orange

2 maraschino cherries

Chocolate Malted Milkshake

The most divinely decadent chocolate milkshake. It's probably worth doubling the quantity, as you are surely going to be asked for refills!

MAKES 2 GLASSES

Two 2-ounce Milky Way bars

1 cup milk

¼ cup Ovaltine malt powder

4 scoops vanilla ice cream

Cut the Milky Way bars into pieces and put into a pan together with the milk and Ovaltine powder. Cook over medium heat, stirring occasionally, until melted. Pour into a bowl or pitcher and let cool. You can speed up the process by placing the container in a bowl of ice. Once it is cool, set aside in the fridge for 1 to 2 hours and then blend together with the vanilla ice cream.

Cookies 'n' Cream Shake

Combine the milk, cookies, and ice cream in a blender and whizz until smooth. Pour into six glasses.

MAKES 6 GLASSES

2 cups milk

6 Oreo cookies, crushed

4 scoops vanilla ice cream

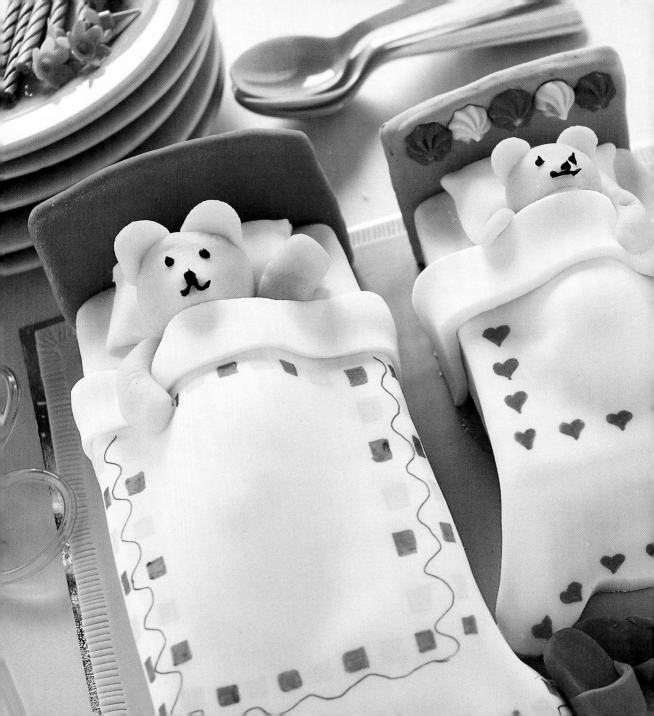

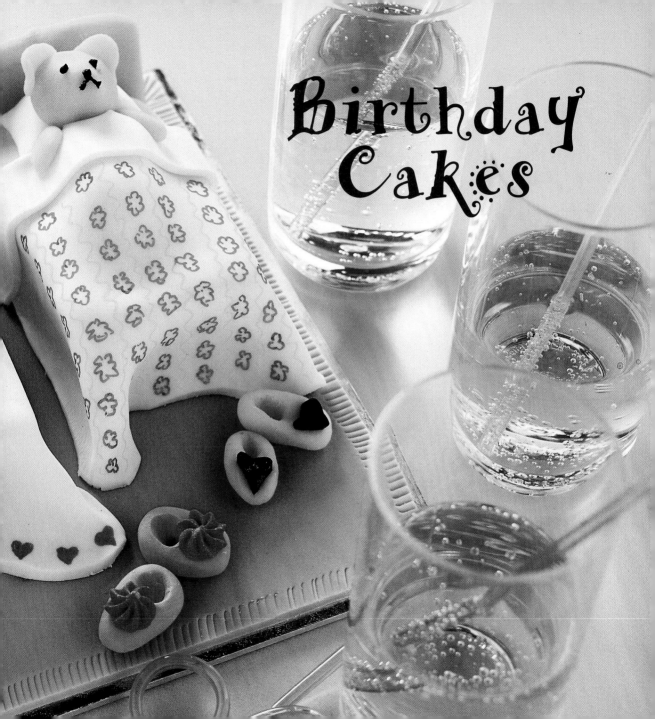

Birthday Cakes

The Three Bears' Cake

SPONGE CAKE

❄ cake before decorating

2 sticks unsalted butter or
   1 tub (8 ounces) soft
   margarine

1 cup superfine sugar

4 large eggs

1½ cups self-rising flour

1 teaspoon pure vanilla extract

½ teaspoon grated lemon zest

DECORATION

One 10 x 14-inch cake board

Strawberry or raspberry jam

1 pound pale blue rolled
   fondant icing (or color white
   fondant blue using a little
   food coloring)

3 tablespoons apricot jam

Overleaf:
The Three Bears' Cake

This is a wonderful cake to make for a young child's birthday. Continue the teddy bear theme of "Goldilocks and the Three Bears" using some of the recipes from the Teddy Bears' Picnic on pages 138–46. You can buy rolled fondant icing at www.wilton.com.

Preheat the oven to 325°F. Lightly grease the base and sides of a 9 x 13-inch cake pan and line with parchment or other baking paper. To make the sponge, cream together the butter and sugar until light and fluffy. Gradually beat in the eggs one at a time, adding 1 tablespoon of the flour with each egg to prevent the mixture from curdling. Beat in the vanilla, the lemon zest, and the remaining flour. Spoon into the prepared pan, level the surface with a spatula, and bake for 30 minutes or until a toothpick inserted in the center comes out clean. Let cool slightly, then turn onto a wire rack, peel off the paper, and let cool completely.

Brush the 10 x 14-inch cake board lightly with strawberry jam. Roll out the pale blue fondant icing thinly and use it to cover the board, trimming the edges and then making a fringe with a sharp knife. Let harden.

TO MAKE THE BUTTERCREAM, cream the butter together with the milk and vanilla and gradually work in the confectioners' sugar. Beat the icing until light and fluffy.

CUT THE SPONGE INTO THREE BEDS of decreasing size (approximately 7 x 4, 5½ x 3, and 4 x 2½ inches). Cut these in half horizontally and sandwich with strawberry jam and buttercream. Arrange the cakes on the board and brush the beds with warmed apricot jam. Roll out the white fondant icing to cover the top third of each bed. Cut out three small rectangles from the remaining sponge cake for pillows and cover each pillow with white fondant icing.

Make torso shapes for each of the teddy bears using the yellow fondant icing and place on the beds. Roll out white fondant bedspreads and drape them over each bed and trim. Add strips of fondant for the turned-down sheets. Shape three bears' heads and paws in decreasing size from yellow fondant icing and decorate their faces with black writing icing. Place a set on each pillow.

CUT OUT THREE HEADBOARDS of decreasing size from heavy cardboard. Brush the headboards with a little warmed apricot jam. Gather the white icing trimmings and divide into two. Color one batch dark blue with a few drops of food coloring and roll out to cover the daddy bear's headboard. Also make him a pair of matching blue slippers. Color the second batch of trimmings pink and roll out to cover the mommy bear's headboard and decorate the top with sugar flowers, sticking them in place with a little jam. Also make a pair of slippers and decorate with sugar flowers. Roll out the remaining yellow icing to cover the baby bear's headboard and make him a pair of matching slippers and decorate with licorice candies.

2¼ pounds white rolled fondant icing
10 ounces yellow rolled fondant icing (or color white icing yellow using a little food coloring)
1 tube black writing icing
Pink and blue food coloring
Sugar flowers
Licorice candies

BUTTERCREAM
1 stick unsalted butter, softened
1 tablespoon milk
½ teaspoon pure vanilla extract
1½ cups confectioners' sugar, sifted

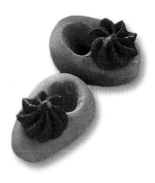

Princess Cake

Butter, for greasing bowl

Flour, for dusting

One 18.25-ounce package
butter recipe golden or
yellow cake mix (Duncan
Hines or Betty Crocker)

FILLING

3 tablespoons raspberry jam

Half a 16-ounce tub vanilla
frosting (Betty Crocker Rich
& Creamy Frosting)

DECORATION

1½ pounds pink rolled fondant
icing

¼ cup apricot jam

6 ounces white rolled fondant
icing

Small round cookie

Candies

Sugar flowers

Mini paper umbrella

Bake this cake in a fairly deep round Pyrex bowl to make the skirt and then cut a hole through the center of the cake and insert the doll. The bowl should be at least 5½ inches deep. In some specialty shops, you can buy a doll decoration that is simply the top half of the doll on a spike. You can buy rolled fondant icing and meringue powder at www.wilton.com.

Preheat the oven to 350°F. Grease a 2.5-quart deep Pyrex bowl with butter and line the base with a circle of waxed paper or baking parchment (this will help the cake turn out of the bowl more easily). Dust the bowl lightly with flour. Prepare the cake mix according to package instructions. Transfer the batter to the Pyrex bowl and bake on the middle rack of the oven for 45 to 50 minutes until the edges of the cake have shrunk away slightly from the edge of the bowl and a toothpick inserted into the center comes out clean.

Remove the cake from the oven and allow to stand for 20 minutes, then turn out onto a wire rack to cool completely (you may need to run a knife around the edge of the bowl to help release the cake). Don't worry if the cake sinks in the center while cooling.

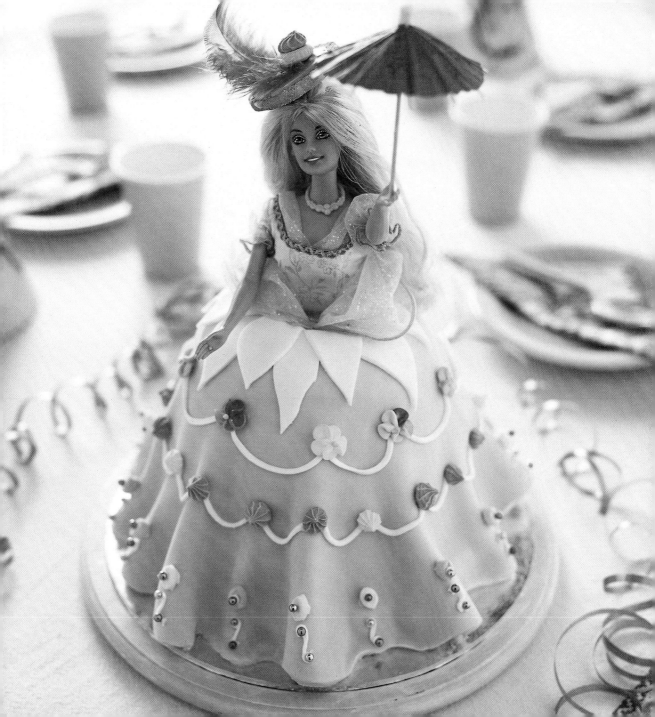

ROYAL ICING

2 cups confectioners' sugar

2½ tablespoons meringue
   powder

When the cake is completely cooled, cut it horizontally into three layers. Place the largest layer top side down on a large plate or cutting board and over it spread two-thirds of the jam followed by two-thirds of the frosting. Put the center layer on top and spread over it the remaining jam and frosting. Finally, put the smallest layer on top, rounded side up. Transfer the sandwiched cake to a cake board.

TO DECORATE, ROLL OUT THE PINK FONDANT into a circle big enough to cover the cake. Warm the apricot jam slightly and brush over the surface of the cake (this will help the fondant stick). Gently lay the fondant over the cake and smooth the top. Ease the fondant down, slightly rippling any excess to look like the folds of a skirt. Trim the bottom with a sharp knife if necessary.

Cut a hole in the top of the cake with a sharp knife. Hollow down through the center until you have a space big enough to fit in a doll. Insert the doll (suitably dressed!) up to her waist. Cut out petals from the white fondant to fill the gap between the doll and the skirt, and if necessary tie a ribbon around her waist or use a band of fondant.

TO MAKE THE ROYAL ICING, put the sugar, meringue powder, and a scant ¼ cup water in the bowl of an electric mixer with the paddle attachment. Mix on low until smooth, about 7 minutes. If the icing is too thick, add a little extra water.

Use the royal icing to pipe lines around the skirt and to attach the candies and sugar flowers as decorations. (Alternatively you could use white writing icing.) Make the doll a hat using a cookie and candy, and attach a feather. Give her an umbrella to hold.

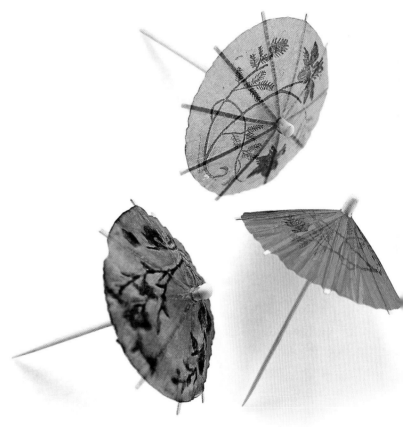

Train Cake

GREEN ICING BASE

5 cups confectioners' sugar

Green food coloring

2 rectangular cake boards
(about 12 x 14 inches)

Green decorating (sanding)
sugar

4 all-butter pound cakes

DECORATION

Melted chocolate or Drizzlers
(for glue)

Blue icing

Yellow icing

Orange icing

Chocolate Twizzlers for railway
track

Black licorice candies

Red Twizzlers for carriage
stripes

Mini Oreos for carriage wheels

Strawberry licorice laces

The good thing about this cake is that it doesn't require any baking. You can make the train as long as you like depending on how many guests you are inviting. Use either spray cans of icing or color frosting in tubs with a little food coloring.

Sift the confectioners' sugar into a large bowl and add ⅓ cup water. Mix to make a spreadable but not runny icing, adding more water if needed. Add the food coloring a little at a time until you have a good green color. Spread the icing over the two cake boards and then sprinkle the decorating sugar on top. Let dry, preferably overnight.

TRIM THE TOPS OFF the pound cakes so that they are flat. To make the engine, make a cut in one of the cakes lengthwise about three-quarters of the way in from one of the long sides. Discard the thinner part of the cake. Make a cut in another cake about two-thirds of the way down from one of the short ends. You should be left with a rectangle of cake about 2¼ inches wide and 5 inches long and a smaller piece about 2¼ inches wide and 2 inches long. Use the smaller piece to make a cab for the engine by setting it on one end of the larger piece of cake, longest side down, and trimming to fit. Attach the cab to the engine using melted chocolate or Drizzlers. Reserve the larger piece.

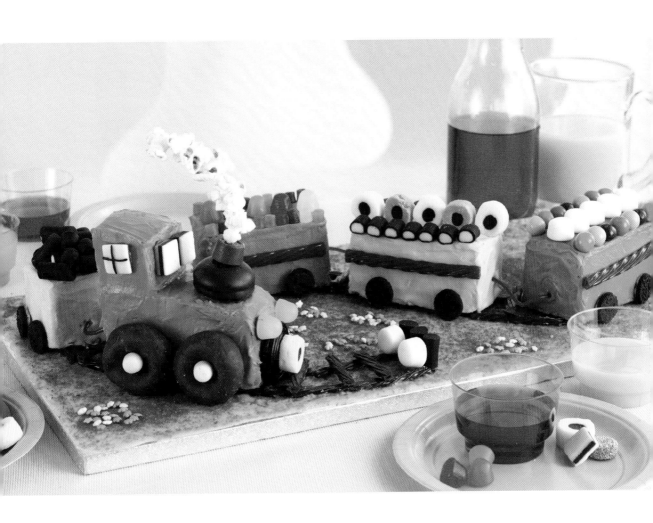

Black licorice wheel

Assorted candies, such as
  gumdrops, jujubes, licorice
  Allsorts

Iced doughnuts for wheels

Popcorn

Thin wire

1 Rolo

1 Mallomar

MAKE CARS from the remaining two cakes by cutting them in the same way as for the engine cab. You should now have three cars about 2¼ inches wide and 5 inches long. Use one of the remaining smaller pieces of cake, 2¼ inches wide and 2 inches long, to make a coal car.

COAT THE ENGINE and one of the cars with blue icing, spreading it evenly all over the cake. Coat the coal car and another car with yellow icing and coat the remaining car with orange icing. Smooth the icing with a wet knife.

Lay out chocolate Twizzlers on the iced cake boards to look like railway track. Slip a spatula underneath the engine and carefully transfer it onto the Twizzler track. Use a table knife to help slide the cake off the spatula. Repeat for the coal car and cars.

Attach the licorice wheel and a candy to the front of the engine to make a fender, using melted chocolate or melted Drizzlers to attach the candies to the cake. Attach yellow gumdrops as headlamps. Use the iced doughnuts as wheels.

To make the funnel and steam, thread six pieces of popcorn onto a piece of wire, leaving a 2-inch piece of wire free. Thread the end of the wire through the center of the Rolo and the center of the Mallomar and then into the engine to secure. *Remove before eating.*

Pile black licorice candies onto the top of the coal car. Decorate the cars with candies and Twizzlers, using blobs of melted chocolate or melted Drizzlers to secure. Use Mini Oreos for wheels. Finally, use licorice laces as couplings to join up the engine and cars.

Swimming Pool Cake

This cake may take a little more time than the others in this book, but it is actually not difficult to make and will certainly make the children want to dive in.

Brush a 10 x 14-inch cake board (or use a slightly larger cake board if you wish) with some warmed apricot jam and position one of the cakes on the board. Cut a 6 x 9-inch rectangle from the center of the second cake.

TO MAKE THE BUTTERCREAM, beat together the butter, sugar, and orange zest and juice until smooth. Spread a thin layer of buttercream over the top of the first cake and place the cake "frame" on top. Reserve a little of the buttercream and use a spatula to cover the cake with the remainder.

TO MAKE THE SWIMMING POOL, use the Belgian chocolate for the decking, cutting it to fit with a long serrated knife in a seesaw action. Sift the sugar into a bowl and beat together with the egg whites or water until thick, then color blue. Reserve a little of the blue icing and spoon or pipe the remainder into the center of the pool, but leave about 1 inch of the inside edge of the pool above the water line and spread this with a thin layer of buttercream.

❄ sponge cake only
2 tablespoons apricot jam
Two 9 x 13-inch sponge cakes
(see Three Bears' Cake on
page 100)

ORANGE BUTTERCREAM
2 sticks unsalted butter,
softened
1 pound sifted confectioners'
sugar
Grated zest and juice of
1 orange

SWIMMING POOL
14 ounces white luxury
Belgian chocolate
1½ cups confectioners' sugar
2 large egg whites or
3 tablespoons water
Blue, pink, brown, yellow, and
red food coloring
8 pink sugar wafers
Colored candies
2 red licorice laces

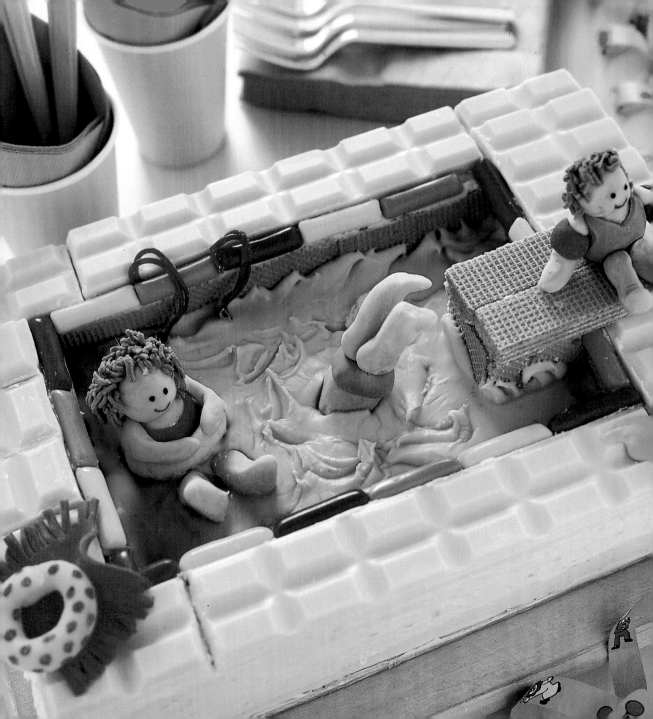

HALVE FIVE PINK WAFERS LENGTHWISE and stick around the inside edge of the pool. Arrange a layer of colored candies above. Use a teaspoon to pull the blue icing to the sides of the pool to look like ripples and make waves on the water's surface. Use the reserved blue icing to make small puddles on the swimming pool deck: These are great for hiding any spaces in the chocolate.

MAKE A DIVING BOARD from a small square cut off from the leftover cake. Stick to the side of the pool with buttercream and cover the top and sides with a thin layer of buttercream. Cover the three sides with halved wafers, cut to fit, and put two whole pink wafers on top. Arrange the licorice laces to form the railings of the steps down to the pool.

FOR THE SWIMMERS, cut the fondant in half and color one half a flesh color. Form into the heads, torsos, and limbs of the swimmers. Color a little of the icing blue, roll on a lightly floured surface, and cut to form bathing trunks and a bathing suit. Color a little red and form into a bathing suit, water wings, and a towel. Color a little brown and push through a garlic press to make hair. Stick onto the swimmers' heads and draw features with icing writers. Color a little yellow and form into two swim tubes. Assemble the swimmers and position as shown in the photograph. Decorate the remaining swim tube with red spots using writing icing and place on top of the towel by the side of the pool.

SWIMMERS
1 pound white rolled
   fondant icing
Food coloring
Black and red writing icing
   pens or tubes of writing
   icing

Burger and Fries

MAKES 10 BURGER AND FRIES
    MEALS

2 pounds white rolled fondant
    icing
Green and red food coloring
Cornstarch
Foil

BURGERS
Three 2-ounce Milky Way bars
1 ounce dark chocolate
6 tablespoons unsalted butter
1 cup Rice Krispies

Decoration ingredients are
    given on page 114

You would have to look twice at these to realize that they are not the real thing! I noticed that at many parties my children attended, a squashed, soggy slice of birthday cake would come back home wrapped in a paper napkin in the party bag. I thought it would be a good idea if the cake wasn't going to be eaten at the party to make really fun-looking individual birthday cakes that the children could take home with them in a little box. These cakes are easy to make and I'm sure older children will love to give you a helping hand.

Use the rolled fondant to make the lettuce leaves first so that they can be molded into shape and left to harden. Cut off 9 ounces (about one-quarter) of the fondant and knead in enough green food coloring to turn it pale green. Roll out into ten thin circles, each approximately 3 inches in diameter, with slightly uneven edges. To make the veins of the lettuce, dip a toothpick into some cornstarch and roll it over the fondant, pressing lightly. Frill the edges of the lettuce by rolling a toothpick dipped in cornstarch backward and forward. Lightly scrunch up ten pieces of foil and form each into circles a little smaller than the lettuce leaves. Lay the green fondant over the foil, press down lightly, and allow to harden overnight.

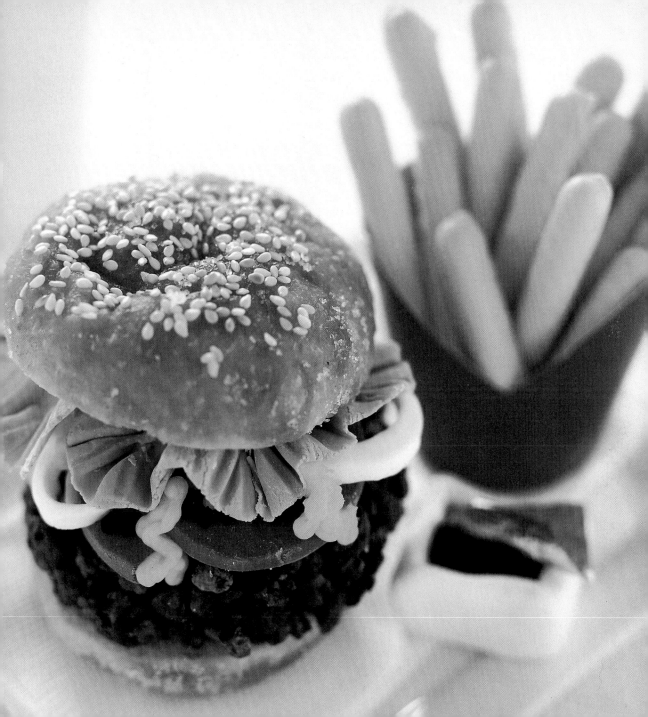

Tubes black and yellow writing
  icing

3 heaping tablespoons
  seedless raspberry jam

3 tablespoons sesame seeds

10 doughnuts about 3 inches
  diameter

10 paper plates

10 red paper cups

Waxed paper

Pound cake cut into "fries"

To make the burgers, cut the Milky Way bars into pieces, put them into a large saucepan together with the chocolate and butter, and melt over low heat, stirring occasionally. Stir in the Rice Krispies until they are well coated. To make the round hamburger shapes, place a 3-inch biscuit cutter on a large nonstick baking pan. Spoon the Rice Krispies mixture into the round biscuit cutter to a depth of about ¼ inch and press down with a teaspoon to level the surface. Carefully remove the biscuit cutter and repeat with the remaining Rice Krispies mixture to make ten burger shapes, and put these in the fridge to set.

For the burger toppings, cut off another 9 ounces of the fondant and color it red by kneading in some red food coloring. Roll out to a thickness of about ¼ inch and cut into ten circles using a 2-inch pastry cutter. Cut each circle in half and use the black writing icing to make little dots of black to resemble the tomato seeds. Cut a slice off the remaining white fondant and form into twenty thin slices of onion.

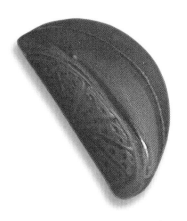

THE TOMATO KETCHUP CONTAINERS are made from the remainder of the white fondant formed into ten small rectangular containers. Fill each of these with 1 teaspoon jam. Add a foil cover, which you can roll back a little to expose the "ketchup." Toast the sesame seeds in a dry frying pan until lightly golden.

TO ASSEMBLE EACH BURGER, cut a doughnut in half horizontally and put one half on a paper plate. Place the Rice Krispies burger on one half, arrange a slice of tomato and two onion slices on top, and pipe on a little yellow writing icing for mustard. Then add a lettuce leaf and place the other half of the doughnut on top and sprinkle with a few of the toasted sesame seeds. Cut about one-third off the height of each red paper cup and cut a V-shape out of the center. Crumple some waxed paper in the base of the cup and arrange about nine pound-cake "fries" in the cup.

PRESENT EACH CHILD with a meal consisting of a burger in a bun, fries, and ketchup. Place on a large paper plate and cover with foil for transporting, or pack into small boxes.

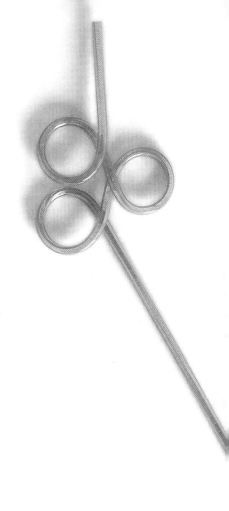

Kitty Cakes

MAKES 6 CATS AND 6 KITTENS

1 package chocolate Drizzlers
9 Twinkies
9 Yodels or Ho Hos
Tubes white and black writing
   icing

DECORATION
White rolled fondant icing
Mini M&M's
Nonpareils
Red licorice laces
Birthday candles

*Turn Twinkies and Yodels into ginger cats and tomcats.
The number of kitties will depend on the age of your
child. Set the tails alight and have the birthday girl or boy
blow them out and make a wish.*

Melt the Drizzlers in the microwave. Use them to make stripes
on six of the Twinkies. Make stripes on six of the Yodels using
white writing icing.

CUT ONE-THIRD OFF EACH END of the un-iced Twinkies and Yodels
to make twelve heads for the cats. Cut circles from the fondant for
the cats' eyes (you can use the top of the writing icing as a guide and
cut around it with a sharp knife, or use the open end of a piping
nozzle) and stick on all the features using some of the melted
Drizzlers (you can stick a toothpick into it, then apply). Add
M&M's for the eyes and draw a vertical line down the center
using black writing icing. Cut the nonpareils into quarters for
the ears and add pink M&M's for the noses and red licorice for
the whiskers.

USE MELTED DRIZZLERS as "glue" to attach the cats' heads
to their bodies. Hold in place until set. Add birthday
candles for tails.

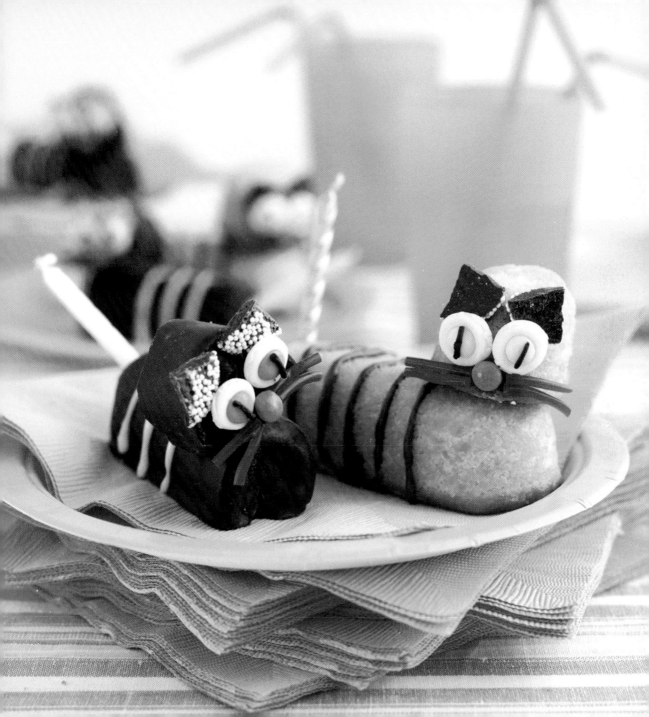

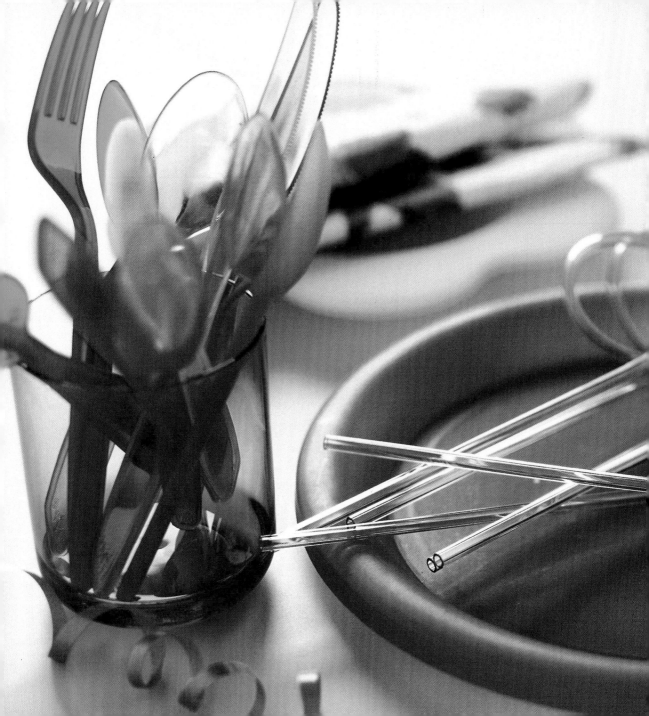

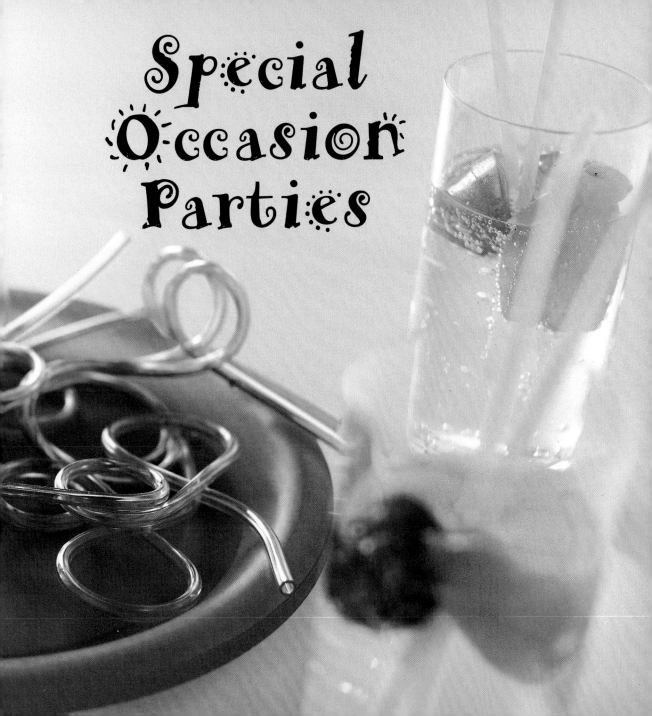

Special Occasion Parties

Easter

EASTER PARTY INVITATIONS
You will need: stiff colored oak tag, colored paper, gold pen (optional), colored ribbons. Cut the oak tag into the shape of an egg and decorate with triangles and strips of colored paper and maybe a gold pen. Write the party details on the back and tie a ribbon with a bow around the middle.

Children love nothing better than a traditional egg hunt. For older children this can involve clues; for younger children, hide the eggs in the yard if the weather is good or around the house. Decorating hard-boiled eggs with paints and glitter or making egg people (see page 125) will keep children amused.

Easter is a chocaholic's dream, but all too often there is a glut of chocolate Easter eggs, so here are a few ideas if you do have surplus stock. Break up hollow Easter eggs to make chocolate chips for use in recipes like Coconut Kisses (page 69) or melt them as in S'mores (page 73). Alternatively, make a fruit fondue by melting chocolate and keeping it warm to use as a dip for a selection of fruits such as strawberries, pineapple, or grapes.

Easter Games

As well as the games featured on pages 18–26, there are some great games specifically to play at Easter.

Easter Egg Hunt

Props: chocolate Easter eggs, baskets or bags. Hide lots of little chocolate Easter eggs around the house or in the yard. Give each child a basket or a bag and let them search and collect as many eggs as they can find. You can give children various tasks like finding eight eggs wrapped in different colors or two wrapped in gold, two wrapped in silver, and two spotted eggs. The winner could get a very special Easter egg as a prize.

Pass the Egg

Props: spoons, chocolate eggs.

Divide the children into two teams. Each child holds a spoon in his or her mouth with the aim of passing a chocolate egg from spoon to spoon without it dropping. If the egg falls on the floor, it has to be picked up with a spoon still held in the mouth.

Spoof!

Props: chocolate mini Easter eggs.

Give the children three Easter eggs each and sit them in a circle. When someone calls "Spoof!," the children have to choose to put none, one, two, or three Easter eggs in their right hand without letting anyone else see how many they have. They should hide their other hand behind their back. The children then take turns guessing the total number of eggs in the children's right hands. For example, if there are six children, there could be as many as eighteen eggs. Jot down the numbers and don't allow anyone to guess the same number as another child. When the children open up their fists, the child who is farthest away from the correct total is out. Keep playing until one child remains.

Chocolate Easter Egg Nests

MAKES 8 CHOCOLATE NESTS

4 ounces milk chocolate

3 ounces dark chocolate

½ stick unsalted butter

3 tablespoons light corn syrup

5 shredded wheat biscuits

Candy-coated mini eggs

Shredded wheat and melted chocolate make perfect nests for candy-coated Easter eggs, which are quick and easy to make.

Break the chocolates into pieces and put into a saucepan together with the butter and corn syrup and melt over low heat. Crush the shredded wheat into a bowl with your fingers.

Line two baking sheets with foil or waxed paper. Stir the shredded wheat into the chocolate mixture and spoon 8 mounds onto the baking sheets, shaping into rounds with dips in the centers.

CHILL IN THE FRIDGE for about an hour until set, then peel off the nests carefully and fill with mini eggs.

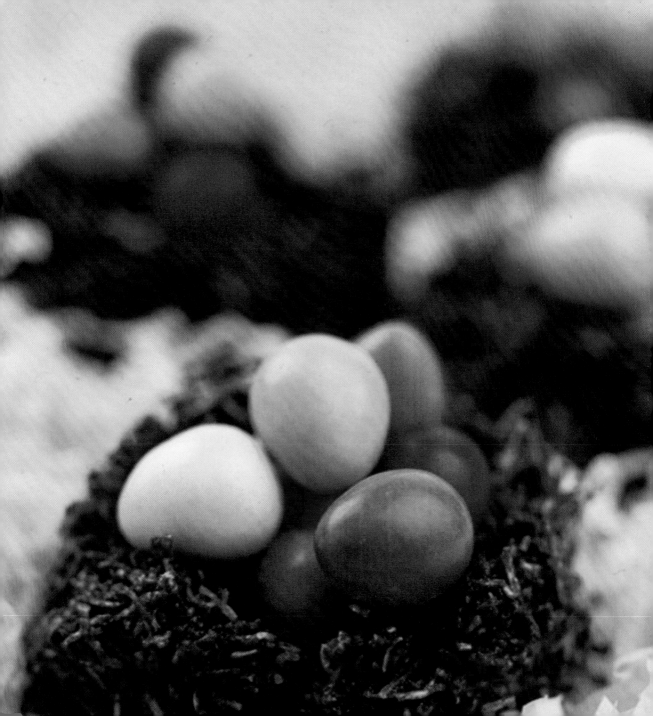

Bunny Cookies

MAKES ABOUT 20 COOKIES

1 recipe for Gingerbread
    Snowflakes (page 193)

DECORATION
Raisins or currants
Mini M&M's, sugar balls, or
    candy-coated chocolate
    beans
Tubes writing icing
Mini marshmallows

These make a great treat. This recipe is fun for older children to make themselves, and they will enjoy cutting out and decorating the cookies. Children can draw their own bunny rabbit shapes, which you can make into oak tag templates to use as guides for cutting out the cookies.

Make the gingerbread cookies, using a bunny cookie cutter.

Once they are cool, decorate with raisins or currants for eyes and mini M&M's, sugar balls, or chocolate beans for buttons, attached with small blobs of writing icing. Draw a nose and whiskers using writing icing. Finish off with a squashed mini marshmallow on the bottom of the cookie for the tail.

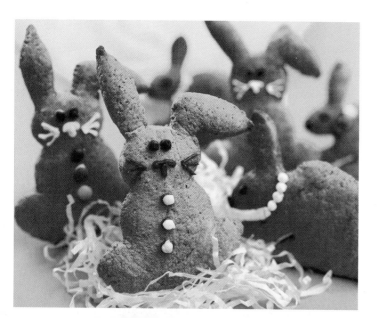

Egg People

A fun activity for children at Easter is to decorate hard-boiled eggs. Make hats from egg cartons, empty toilet paper rolls, and odds and ends like feathers, cotton balls, lace, and ribbon. You can make braids from yarn and paint faces on the eggs with black and red felt-tip pens.

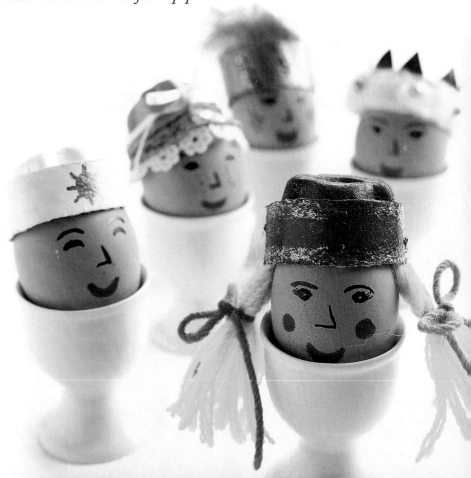

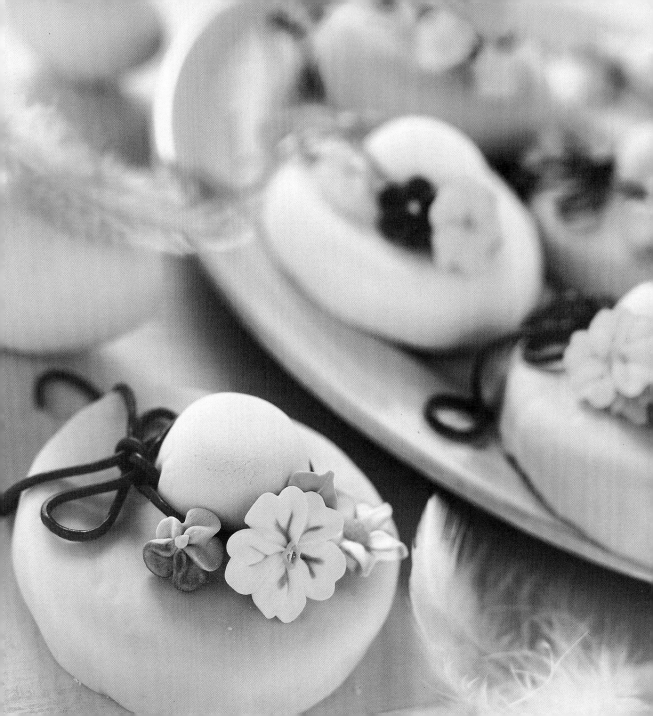

Easter Bonnet Cakes

These are easy to make and look fabulous. You can color the icing using a few drops of food coloring to make different-colored hats.

Preheat the oven to 350°F. Cream together the butter and sugar until light and fluffy. Add an egg at a time, each with 1 tablespoon of the flour. Fold in the remaining flour together with the milk, lemon zest, and vanilla.

Grease and flour two 9 x 13-inch shallow baking pans. Spread the batter evenly over the base of the pans and bake for 20 minutes (a toothpick inserted in the center of the cake will come out clean when the cake is ready).

TO MAKE THE BONNETS, cut each cake into six circles using a 3-inch round cutter. Stick a marshmallow in the center of each circle using warmed apricot jam. Roll out 2 ounces of fondant at a time and cut into circles about 1½ inches wider than the cakes all the way around. Brush the marshmallows and cake bases with warmed apricot jam and lay the circles of fondant over the centers. Mold to the shapes of the cakes and trim away any excess fondant. Tie licorice laces in a bow around the bases of the marshmallows and decorate with sugar flowers, attaching them to the fondant with a little of the warmed apricot jam.

MAKES 12 EASTER BONNET CAKES

1 stick plus 2 tablespoons unsalted butter

¾ cup superfine sugar

3 large eggs

1 cup plus 2 tablespoons self-rising flour

1 tablespoon milk

½ teaspoon grated lemon zest

1 teaspoon pure vanilla extract

12 marshmallows

¼ cup apricot jam

1½ pounds white rolled fondant icing

DECORATION

Red and green licorice laces

Sugar flowers

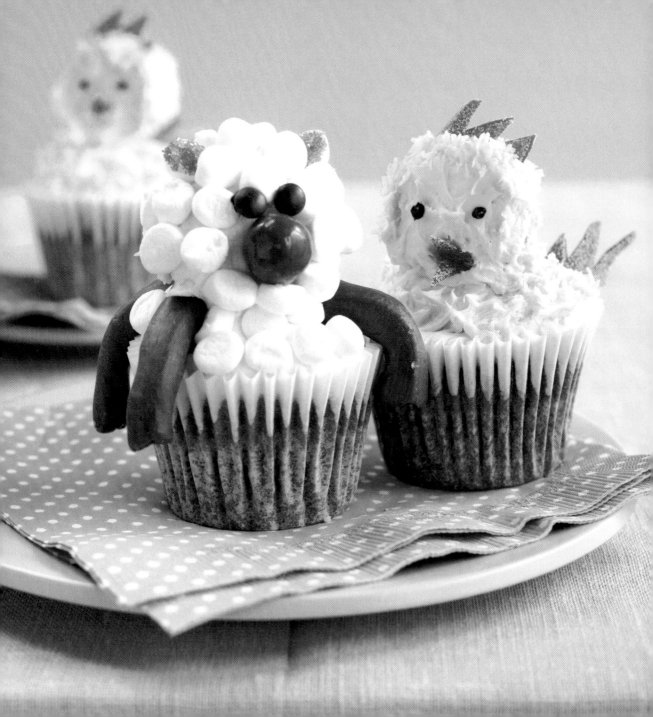

Easter Cupcake Animals

Preheat the oven to 350°F. Line a standard muffin pan and a mini muffin pan with paper liners. Prepare the cake mix according to package instructions. Fill the muffin cups. Bake the minis for about 15 minutes and the larger cupcakes for about 25 minutes. Remove from the pans and let cool in their liners.

To DECORATE THE CHICKS, tint the frosting yellow and ice the tops of 6 large cupcakes. Remove the liners from 6 minis and ice the tops and sides. Tint the coconut yellow. Roll the minis in the coconut and place on top of each large cupcake. Draw eyes with black icing. Ice the back and cover it and the top of the large cupcake with coconut. Make combs and beaks from the fruit leather.

To DECORATE THE SHEEP, ice the tops of 6 large cupcakes. Cut the marshmallows in half using scissors. For ears, dip 12 marshmallow halves, cut side down, into the sugar and set aside. Arrange marshmallows on top of the cupcakes, leaving enough space in the center for a mini. Remove the liners from 6 minis and ice the tops and sides. Use a malted milk ball for the nose, and attach the ears. Place a mini on its side on top of each large cupcake; ice the back and cover with marshmallows. Use M&M's for eyes. Place two Tootsie Rolls on each side of the cupcake for legs.

MAKES 12 CUPCAKES

One 18.25-ounce box devil's food cake mix (Duncan Hines or Betty Crocker)

One 16-ounce tub vanilla frosting (Betty Crocker Rich & Creamy Frosting)
Yellow food coloring
⅔ cup sweetened flaked coconut
1 tube black writing icing
Red fruit leather

One 16-ounce tub vanilla frosting (Betty Crocker Rich & Creamy Frosting)
Mini marshmallows
Pink decorating sugar
6 malted milk balls
12 brown mini M&M's or other mini candies
24 mini Tootsie Rolls

Mother's Day Breakfast

This is always on a Sunday, so it is a perfect opportunity for children to do something really special for their mother—or father on Father's Day. Children will adore presenting their mom or dad with an indulgent breakfast in bed. For young children, Dad can lend a hand on Mother's Day and Mom can help out on Father's Day. If Dad is partial to a cooked breakfast, you could help your child prepare the heart-shaped egg on page 135 and serve it with bacon or sausages.

Apart from the recipes themselves, you can go to town on the presentation. Lay a pretty napkin over a tray and maybe put a single rose in a small vase. Perhaps write and design a breakfast menu and don't forget to include Mom or Dad's favorite newspaper or magazine and a nice cup of tea or coffee. Post a note on the fridge door the night before telling Mom or Dad to sleep in the following morning and to expect breakfast in bed. Alternatively, make it a big surprise—but you will need to get out of bed early!

Buttermilk Pancakes

These pancakes can be made in advance, refrigerated, and reheated. Pancakes also freeze well. Interleave with waxed paper, then wrap in a freezer bag and freeze for up to a month. Thaw at room temperature for several hours.

Sift the flour, baking powder, and salt into a large bowl. Stir in the sugar. Make a well in the center of the flour and pour in the egg. Use a wooden spoon to gradually stir the flour into the egg, adding the buttermilk a little at a time, until you have a smooth batter. Stir in 1 tablespoon of the melted butter and transfer the batter to a pitcher.

PUT A HEAVY SKILLET over medium heat and grease with a little of the melted butter. Pour about 2 tablespoons batter into the pan and cook for 1½ to 2 minutes until the surface is covered with small bubbles and the underside is golden brown. Use a spatula to flip the pancake over and cook for 1 minute or until light brown. Lift the cooked pancake out of the skillet with the spatula. Regrease the skillet and continue to cook the pancakes until all the batter has been used up. To keep the pancakes warm, transfer them on a plate to a low oven, about 200°F. Serve with berries and maple syrup.

MAKES 6 PANCAKES

1 cup all-purpose flour

1 teaspoon baking powder

Large pinch of salt

1 tablespoon superfine sugar

1 large egg, lightly beaten

¾ cup buttermilk

3 tablespoons unsalted butter, melted

1 cup berries, for serving

Maple syrup, for serving

Fruit Salad with Honey Yogurt Dressing

Fresh fruit presented in a slightly different way makes a great treat for Mom. Make a fruit salad using seasonal fruits and top with a mixture of plain yogurt and honey. Alternatively, make a fruit plate and serve with a bowl of yogurt and honey for dipping.

Mango, Strawberry, and Banana Fruit Smoothie

MAKES 1 TALL OR 2 SMALL GLASSES

3 strawberries

½ cup peeled and chopped mango

1 small or ½ medium banana

Juice of 1 orange

1 passion fruit (optional)

This is especially good when sweet, juicy mangoes are in season. You could also make this using a fresh juicy peach instead of banana when peaches are in season.

Wash and hull the strawberries and then simply blend all the fruit together.

Apple and Carrot Breakfast Muffins

Here is a healthy and deliciously moist muffin that's bound to become a family favorite. These muffins are very easy to make and will keep well for up to five days.

Preheat the oven to 350°F. Combine the flour, sugar, powdered milk, baking powder, cinnamon, salt, and ginger in a mixing bowl. In a separate bowl, combine the oil, honey, maple syrup, eggs, and vanilla. Beat lightly with a wire whisk until blended. Add the apple, carrot, and raisins to the liquid mixture and stir well. Fold in the dry ingredients until just combined, but don't overmix, or the muffins will become heavy. Line a muffin pan with paper liners and fill the muffin cups two-thirds full. Bake for 20 to 25 minutes.

MAKES 12 MUFFINS

1 cup whole-wheat flour

¼ cup sugar

2 tablespoons nonfat dry milk

1½ teaspoons baking powder

½ teaspoon ground cinnamon

¼ teaspoon salt

¼ teaspoon ground ginger

½ cup canola oil

¼ cup honey

¼ cup maple syrup

2 large eggs, lightly beaten

½ teaspoon pure vanilla extract

1 large apple, peeled and
    grated

½ cup grated carrot

½ cup raisins

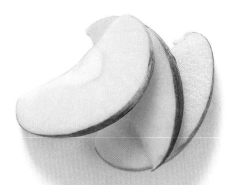

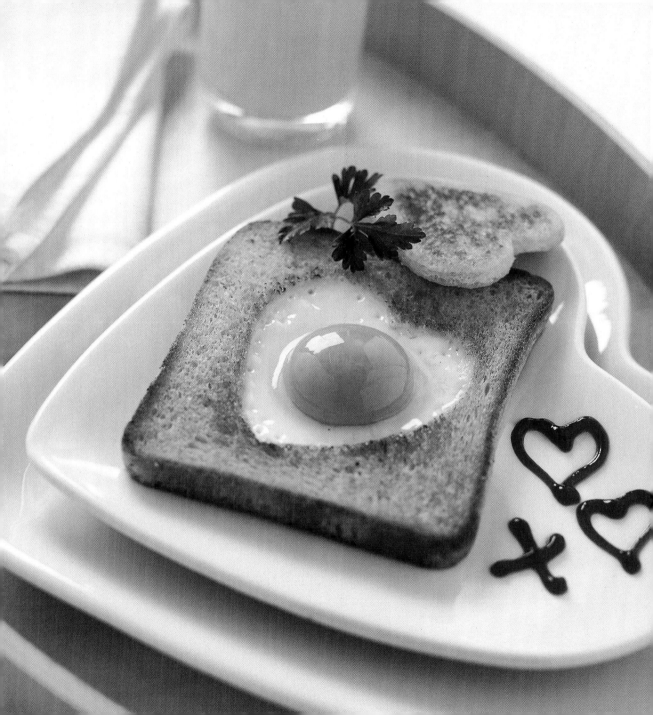

A Hearty Breakfast

This heart-shaped egg would make a fun surprise breakfast for Mom or Dad and only takes a few minutes to prepare. It would be fun also to pipe Mommy or Daddy's name on the plate using some ketchup—this can be done using a pastry bag with a thin nozzle, or you can make your own throwaway pastry bag by rolling up a small piece of waxed paper. Older children will enjoy helping you make this.

Cut a hole in the center of the bread using a heart-shaped cookie cutter about 3 inches wide at its widest point. Melt the 1 tablespoon butter in a small frying pan and sauté the bread on one side until golden. Turn the bread over, melt the extra pat of butter in the heart-shaped cutout, break the egg into it, and season lightly. Cook covered for about 2 minutes until the egg is cooked to Mom's or Dad's liking. You can also dip the cutout heart in a little egg and sauté that, too, to make French toast.

SERVES 1

1 thick slice white bread

1 tablespoon unsalted butter
    plus an extra pat

1 large Eggland's Best
    egg

Salt and freshly ground black
    pepper

Mock Fried Egg

SERVES 1

1 small container vanilla or
   plain yogurt
1 fresh or canned peach half

You would have to look closely at this to see that it is a no-cholesterol version of a fried egg!

Carefully spoon the yogurt into a colored bowl or plate and then place the peach half rounded side up in the center to look like the yolk.

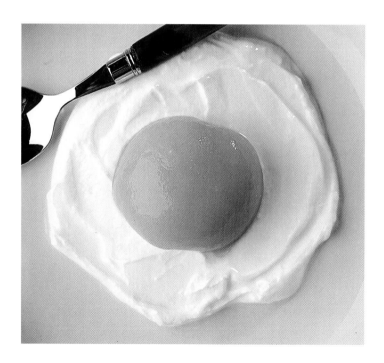

Toasted Ham and Cheese Muffin

Toasted English muffins make a great base for all sorts of toppings, such as creamy scrambled eggs. You can add extras like grated cheese and chopped tomatoes or snipped chives.

Preheat the broiler. Split the muffin, arrange the two halves upside down on a broiling pan, and broil for 1 minute. Remove, turn over, and spread with a little butter. Divide the ham between the two halves and add the Worcestershire sauce. Top with grated cheese and broil for 3 to 4 minutes until golden.

SERVES 1

1 English muffin
Butter or margarine
2 wafer-thin slices ham
Few drops of Worcestershire sauce
¼ cup grated Cheddar or Swiss cheese

Tuna Melt

This is quick and easy to make and tastes delicious.

Drain and flake the tuna. Mix together with the ketchup, yogurt or crème fraîche, and scallions. Split the muffins and toast them. Spread with the tuna mixture and sprinkle with the grated Cheddar. Place the muffins under the broiler and broil until the cheese is golden and bubbling.

SERVES 2

One 6-ounce can tuna in oil or water
2 tablespoons ketchup
1 tablespoon yogurt or crème fraîche
1 or 2 finely sliced scallions
2 English muffins
⅓ cup grated Cheddar cheese

Teddy Bears' Picnic

TEDDY BEARS' PICNIC INVITATIONS

You will need: colored sheets of 8½ x 11-inch paper, cellophane tape, envelopes, pencil, felt-tip pens.

Take two sheets of paper. Fold each sheet in half to make it 5½ x 8½ inches and then fold in half again so that it is 2¾ inches wide. Draw a teddy bear on the paper about 5 inches tall with the teddy bear's arms open quite wide and stretching right to the edges of the paper. Cut around the outline of the teddy bear, but do not cut around the folded edges. Unfold the bears and stick together the two strips of paper with cellophane tape, and you will have eight teddy bears holding hands. Draw faces on the teddy bears and write the party details on the back.

A teddy bear picnic is fun, particularly in the summer when you can hold it outdoors. You don't even have to venture far, as it can be just as much fun in your own backyard. However, always have an alternative indoor venue if the weather turns against you—even if it is only a large rug on the kitchen floor.

Adding to the Fun

- Ask each child to bring along a favorite teddy bear.
- As a fun activity, get the children to make up Edible Necklaces (page 145) when they arrive, which they can either wear around their necks or adorn their teddy bears with.
- Make up the picnic so that you can give each child an individual box of food containing sandwiches, cakes, fruit, etc.
- After the picnic, make up clues so the children can go on a treasure hunt for the "honeypot" filled with lots of goodies.
- Wash fruit thoroughly before packing it up for the picnic so that it is ready to eat as soon as you get there.

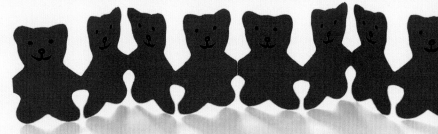

Teddy Bears' Picnic Games

As well as the games featured on pages 18–26, here are some ideas for games to play at a teddy bears' picnic.

Treasure Hunt

Props: cream-colored paper, matches, pen.

Before the picnic, write and hide clues. Give out the first clue, which will lead to the second, third, and eventually the treasure. It is fun to write the clues on sheets of paper that have been singed around the edges with a match and then rolled up and tied with string. Another way to hide clues is to write them on a small piece of paper, insert them into a balloon, then blow up the balloon and hide it. To read the clue, the children will first have to burst the balloon.

"Teddy says . . ."

Prop: one teddy bear.

Holding a teddy, stand in front of the children and make up actions such as "Teddy says hop on one foot." All the children have to hop on one foot until he decides to change the action to something such as, "Teddy says touch your nose with your foot." The catch is that the action must be prefixed by "Teddy says" for them to follow orders. If he says, "Go on all fours and bark like a dog," the children should not follow because Teddy didn't say so. Any child who does the action by mistake is then out. The game continues until only one child is left.

WHAT TO TAKE ON A PICNIC

A plastic sheet to put on the ground.

Rugs to sit on.

Plenty of paper napkins or paper towels and maybe some wet wipes.

Ice packs and an insulated bag for keeping drinks and food cold.

Paper plates and plastic cups.

Plastic cartons for transporting salads and sandwiches, etc.

Some large plastic trash bags to put all the trash in.

Leafy green salads packed separately from the dressing so they don't go mushy.

Small prizes for the games.

Salad on a Stick

Cubes or slices of cheese

Chunks of cucumber and
carrot

Cherry tomatoes

Turkey slices

Seedless grapes

Pineapple chunks

Kiwi slices

Strawberries

Dried apricots

Barbecued chicken chunks

Ham slices

Serve a variety of healthy foods on a wooden skewer. Make savory kebabs or fruit kebabs using any of the suggestions given here.

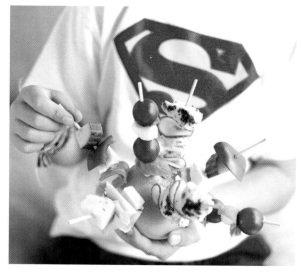

Teddy Bear Sandwiches

It's fun to make sandwiches cut into teddy bear shapes using cookie cutters. Choose some popular fillings for the sandwiches such as peanut butter, cream cheese, or strawberry jam. If you find teddy bear cookie cutters in varying sizes, you can even make a family of teddy bears.

Chocolate-Orange Mini Cupcakes

Mini cupcakes are just the right size for small children, and these are really easy and quick to make. The combination of chocolate with a hint of orange is irresistible.

Preheat the oven to 350°F. Cream together the butter and superfine sugar. Sift together the flour and cocoa. Add the eggs to the creamed mixture, a little at a time, together with 1 tablespoon of the flour mixture. Fold in the remaining flour and cocoa until blended. Stir in the orange zest and chocolate chips. Line some muffin pans with paper liners and fill each of the liners two-thirds full. Transfer to the oven and bake for 12 to 15 minutes. When cool, sieve some confectioners' sugar over the cupcakes for decoration, if you like.

ALTERNATIVELY, decorate to look like teddy bears using chocolate buttons for ears and mini M&M's for the eyes and nose, stuck on with melted chocolate. Use red writing icing for the mouth.

MAKES 30 MINI CUPCAKES

❄ without the decoration

1 stick unsalted butter or
  ½ cup soft margarine
½ cup superfine sugar
1 cup self-rising flour
2 tablespoons Dutch-process
  cocoa powder
2 large eggs, lightly beaten
Grated zest of 1 small orange
½ cup chocolate chips
Confectioners' sugar (optional)

DECORATION
Chocolate buttons
Mini M&M's
Melted chocolate
1 tube red writing icing

OVERLEAF: Teddy Bear Sandwiches (see left), Chocolate-Orange Mini Cupcakes (see above), Teddy Bear Cookies (page 144)

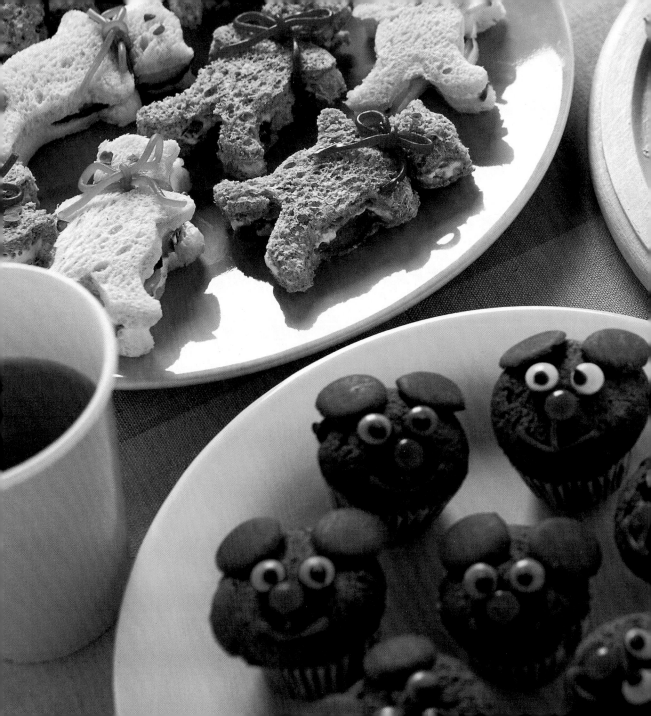

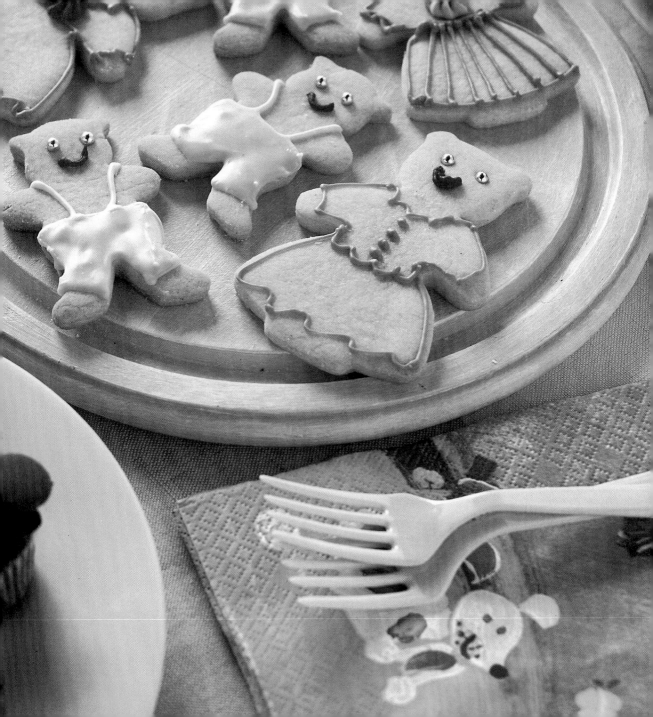

Teddy Bear Cookies

MAKES 20 COOKIES

❄ without the decoration

1 stick unsalted butter,
    at room temperature

¼ cup superfine sugar

1 cup plus 2 tablespoons
    all-purpose flour

Pinch of salt

Few drops of pure
    vanilla extract

DECORATION

Edible silver balls or currants
    or raisins

Glacé Icing (see page 66)

Pink and blue food coloring

Sugar flowers

Thin ribbon (optional)

Children love these teddy-bear-shaped cookies, and they are easy and quick to make. I have various-size teddy bear cookie cutters, so I can make a whole family of teddy bears.

Preheat the oven to 350°F. Beat the butter and sugar together either by hand with a wooden spoon or in an electric mixer. Sift together the flour and salt and mix this into the butter mixture together with a few drops of vanilla to form a fairly stiff dough. If the dough is too dry, add a little water. Form the dough into a ball, then roll out thinly on a floured work surface using a rolling pin dusted with flour. Cut into teddy shapes using cookie cutters. Collect all the trimmings together and roll these out again to make more cookies. Add silver balls or currants for eyes before baking. Bake for about 15 minutes until the cookies are lightly golden. Cool the cookies on a wire rack.

MAKE UP ONE RECIPE OF THE GLACÉ ICING and color one-half pink and one-half pale blue. Pipe clothes onto the teddy bears using the icing and decorate some of the girl teddies with sugar flowers. Alternatively, leave the teddy bears plain and tie bows of thin ribbon around their necks.

Edible Necklaces

Making necklaces using an assortment of non-messy foods is great fun for children. Use a large, fairly blunt needle and choose from the listed foods to design your own necklace on a length of yarn or use licorice laces. A good way to encourage your child to eat healthy foods is to thread two or three treats onto the necklace after the healthy foods so that your child has to eat the healthy foods before reaching the treats.

Yarn or licorice laces

HEALTHY FOODS

Miniature cheeses

Chunks of cucumber, carrot, celery, or bell pepper

Cherry tomatoes

Dried apricots and apple rings

Dates

Breakfast cereals with holes in the middle

Round pretzels

Purple, red, and green grapes

TREATS

Licorice Allsorts

Marshmallows

Life Savers

Cookies with holes in the middle

Combos

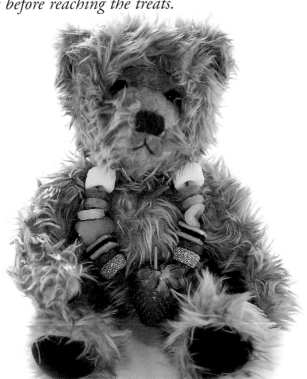

Chicken Salad

SERVES 6

2 cups chicken stock

2 small chicken breasts, cut into bite-size pieces

4 ounces pasta shapes, cooked and cooled

1⅓ cups canned or cooked frozen corn, drained

18 small cherry tomatoes, cut in half

2 scallions, finely sliced

Shredded romaine lettuce

DRESSING

3 tablespoons olive oil

1 tablespoon white wine vinegar

½ teaspoon Dijon mustard

½ teaspoon sugar

Salt and freshly ground black pepper

1 tablespoon chicken stock from the poaching liquid

This is a delicious, easy-to-prepare chicken salad. You could substitute flaked tuna for the chicken if you like.

Poach the chicken for 10 minutes in the stock, then let cool completely. Remove the chicken with a slotted spoon, reserving the poaching liquid. This can be done the night before. To make the dressing, whisk together all of the ingredients (or use a hand blender). Mix together all of the salad ingredients and toss in the dressing.

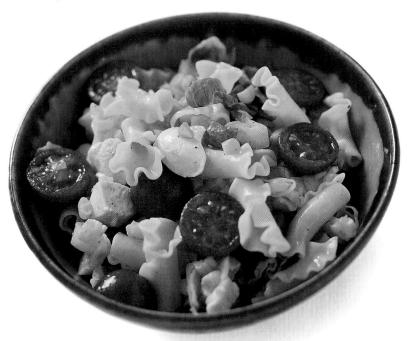

Fourth of July

Summer barbecues are always great fun, and it's a good opportunity to get Dad involved in the cooking.

Organize any of the outdoor games on pages 25 and 26, and make sure the children are well away from the barbecue.

For a Fourth of July celebration, it's fun to keep all the tableware in patriotic red, white, and blue combinations. Red checkered tablecloths look great.

It's easy to make your own invitations. Stick a white card onto a red border. Design your own flag and decorate with red and blue stickers. Write your party details in red and blue markers on the back.

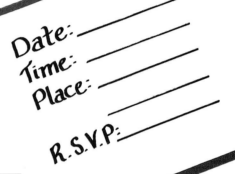

Date: _____
Time: _____
Place: _____

R.S.V.P: _____

You're Invited,
To Our
Fourth of July Party

Sticky Drumsticks

MAKES 6 DRUMSTICKS

6 large chicken drumsticks

MARINADE

2 teaspoons soy sauce

2 teaspoons Worcestershire
   sauce

¼ cup ketchup

2 tablespoons Chinese plum
   sauce

2 tablespoons dark brown
   sugar

½ teaspoon Dijon mustard

A good way to marinate drumsticks is to put the marinade in a clean plastic food or freezer bag, add the drumsticks, seal the top tightly, and rub the sauce and chicken together. Leave the bag in the fridge for at least an hour. You can buy Chinese plum sauce in most supermarkets— it adds a delicious flavor to these drumsticks.

Score the drumsticks three times with a sharp knife. Mix together all the ingredients for the marinade. Marinate the drumsticks for at least 1 hour or overnight. Transfer to a baking dish and baste well. Preheat the broiler and cook the drumsticks for about 20 minutes or until cooked through, turning occasionally and basting with the barbecue sauce.

CHECK THAT THE DRUMSTICKS ARE COOKED THROUGH, wrap the ends in foil, and serve with baked beans and baked potatoes. Alternatively, cook the drumsticks in an oven preheated to 375°F for 35 to 40 minutes.

Pinwheel Pizzas

These pizzas are just the right size for little fingers. They also make tasty morsels for the grown-ups and look much more attractive than pizza slices. If you don't want to make your own pastry, make the crust with frozen pastry.

Sift together the flour and salt. Using your fingertips, rub in the butter so that the mixture resembles fine bread crumbs. Stir in the grated cheese and dried herbs. Stir in the milk until the mixture forms a soft dough. Turn onto a lightly floured surface and knead for 1 minute or until smooth (don't knead for too long, as the dough becomes greasy).

Roll out the dough on a sheet of waxed paper to a rectangle of about 12 x 8 inches. Sauté the onion and mushrooms in the olive oil for 3 to 4 minutes. Stir in the pesto and tomato puree. Spread the mushroom and tomato mixture over the rolled-out dough and sprinkle the grated cheese on top.

PREHEAT THE OVEN TO 350°F. To create the pinwheel effect, use the waxed paper as a guide and roll up the dough from the long side. Remove the waxed paper and, using a sharp knife, cut into about 12 slices, each about ¾ inch thick. Place cut side down on a greased baking pan and bake for about 20 minutes until golden.

MAKES ABOUT 12 INDIVIDUAL
PINWHEEL PIZZAS

❄

1½ cups self-rising flour

¼ teaspoon salt

½ stick unsalted butter

½ cup grated Cheddar cheese

1 teaspoon Italian seasoning

½ cup milk

TOPPING

1 medium onion, chopped

1 cup button mushrooms, chopped

1 tablespoon olive oil

2 tablespoons red pesto

2 tablespoons tomato puree or sauce

1 cup grated Cheddar cheese

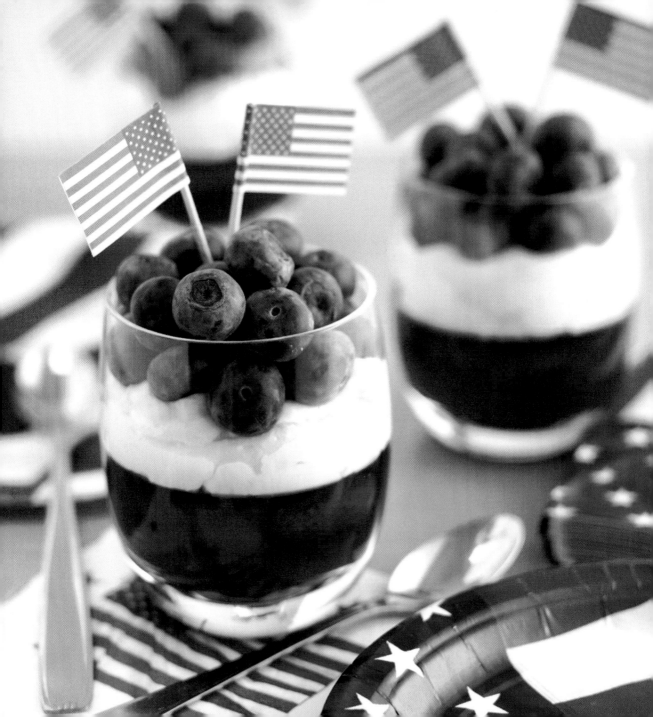

Red, White, and Blueberry Sundaes

An easy to prepare but very popular dessert. You can make the gelatin in advance and then finish off with the whipped cream, meringue, and fresh berries.

Divide the strawberries among four glasses. Prepare the gelatin according to the package instructions and pour over the strawberries. Place in the fridge until set.

WHIP THE CREAM. Break the meringues into pieces and stir into the whipped cream. When the gelatin is set, divide the cream among the four glasses.

SPOON A LAYER OF BLUEBERRIES on top and decorate with the U.S. flag.

MAKES 4 GLASSES

6 large strawberries, hulled
   and quartered
One 3-ounce package
   cranberry-raspberry gelatin
   dessert (or another red
   flavor)
1 cup heavy cream
2 meringue nests
1 cup blueberries

DECORATION
Mini U.S. flags

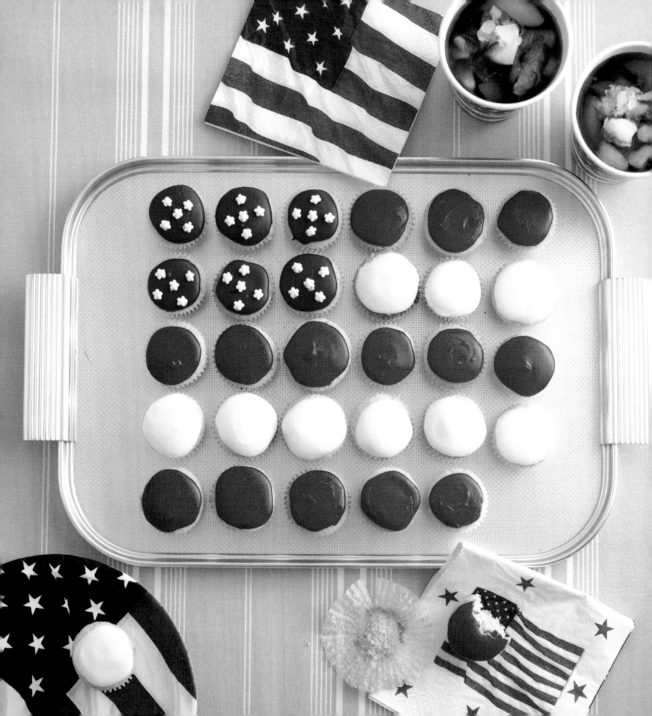

Stars and Stripes Mini Cupcakes

So simple but really effective. You can make this with the vanilla cupcake mixture below or leave out the vanilla and stir in 2 tablespoons Dutch-process cocoa powder, ½ cup chocolate chips, and the grated zest of ½ orange and have delicious chocolate-orange cupcakes.

Preheat the oven to 350°F. Put all the cupcake ingredients into a bowl or food processor and beat together until smooth. Line a mini muffin pan with paper liners and fill each liner about two-thirds full with the batter. Bake for 10 to 12 minutes until well risen and the cakes spring back when you press them with your fingertips.

MIX THE SUGAR WITH 3½ to 4 tablespoons warm water until you have a good spreadable consistency—it should not be runny. You may need to add a little extra water. Remove 1½ tablespoons of the icing and color it blue. Remove two-thirds of the remaining icing and color it red.

ICE SIX OF THE CUPCAKES BLUE, fifteen of the cupcakes red, and nine of the cupcakes white. Stick white sugar stars on the blue-iced cupcakes and arrange the mini cupcakes in the design of the American flag.

MAKES ABOUT 36 MINI CUPCAKES
(you will use 30 for the flag)

1 stick unsalted butter or
 ½ cup soft margarine
½ cup superfine sugar
1 cup self-rising flour
2 large eggs
1 teaspoon pure vanilla extract

GLACÉ ICING
2 cups confectioners' sugar
Blue and red food coloring

DECORATION
Mini white sugar stars or
 piped white icing stars

Sticky Ribs

SERVES 4

3 pounds spareribs, cut into
  individual ribs
Salt and freshly ground black
  pepper
Paprika

BBQ SAUCE
1 tablespoon white wine
  vinegar
2 teaspoons soy sauce
¼ cup light brown sugar
½ cup ketchup
½ teaspoon Dijon mustard
1 tablespoon Worcestershire
  sauce
1 clove garlic, crushed
Salt and freshly ground black
  pepper

The Fourth of July is generally a barbecue event and these sticky ribs always make popular barbecue food.

Season the ribs with salt, pepper, and paprika. Grill over medium heat for 10 minutes on each side. Meanwhile mix together all the ingredients for the BBQ sauce.

Brush the BBQ sauce thickly over the ribs, turn, and cook for 4 to 5 minutes. Turn again. Repeat three to four times until the ribs are cooked through and sticky. Total cooking time will probably be 40 minutes (20 minutes without the BBQ sauce plus 20 minutes cooking with basting).

YOU CAN ALSO COOK THE RIBS IN THE OVEN. Line a roasting pan with a large piece of foil, toss the ribs in the BBQ sauce, and arrange on the foil. Cover the pan with another piece of foil and bake for 30 minutes at 325°F. Uncover the pan and bake for a further 20 to 30 minutes at 400°F. Cool slightly before serving.

Barbecue Baked Potatoes

Wash and dry the potatoes, prick the skins several times, and brush with oil. Either place directly on the grill or wrap each potato in aluminum foil and cook for 45 to 60 minutes, turning occasionally, depending on the size of the potato. They are delicious if you scoop out the flesh, leaving a shell, and mash together with some butter, sour cream, snipped chives, and seasoning. Spoon the mixture back into the shell and heat through on the barbecue.

Baking potatoes

Canola oil

Butter

Sour cream

Fresh chives

Salt and freshly ground black
   pepper

Corn on the Cob

Remove the husks and silk and rinse the corn well. Place each cob on a sheet of extra thick aluminum foil. Brush all over with the softened butter. Season with salt and pepper and sprinkle with water. Fold over the foil to make a snug package. Place on the barbecue and grill for 20 minutes or until the corn is tender, turning several times. Unwrap the corn, taking care, as it will be very hot, and barbecue for a couple of minutes, turning occasionally to get a slightly charred effect. For young children it is best to cut the cobs in half before they are barbecued.

SERVES 4

4 ears of corn

1 tablespoon butter, softened

Salt and freshly ground black
   pepper

Teriyaki Chicken Burgers

MAKES 8 BURGERS

1 onion, finely chopped

½ red bell pepper, cored,
    seeded, and chopped

1 tablespoon canola oil

½ chicken bouillon cube

1 apple, peeled, grated, and
    squeezed to drain

¾ pound chicken breast,
    roughly chopped, or

¾ pound lean ground beef

1 tablespoon chopped fresh
    parsley

¼ cup fresh white bread crumbs

Salt and freshly ground
    black pepper

TERIYAKI SAUCE

3 tablespoons soy sauce

1½ teaspoons sesame oil

3 tablespoons sake

3 tablespoons mirin
    (sweet rice wine)

1 tablespoon superfine sugar

Here are tasty burgers that can be cooked on a barbecue or under the broiler. I have given a recipe for making your own teriyaki sauce, but as a shortcut you could use a store-bought teriyaki sauce. The homemade teriyaki sauce would make a good marinade for the beef or chicken skewers featured on pages 158 and 159.

Sauté the onion and bell pepper in the oil until softened. Dissolve the bouillon cube in 3 tablespoons boiling water. Put all the ingredients for the burgers into a food processor, including the onion and bell pepper, and chop for a few seconds. Using floured hands, form the mixture into eight burgers.

To make the sauce, put the ingredients into a small saucepan, bring to a boil, then reduce the heat and simmer for about 2 minutes until slightly thickened and reduced by half. Place the burgers directly on the grill or use a hinged basket, which holds the food between two wire racks. Grill or barbecue for 4 minutes on one side, then baste with the sauce and cook for another minute. Repeat on the other side.

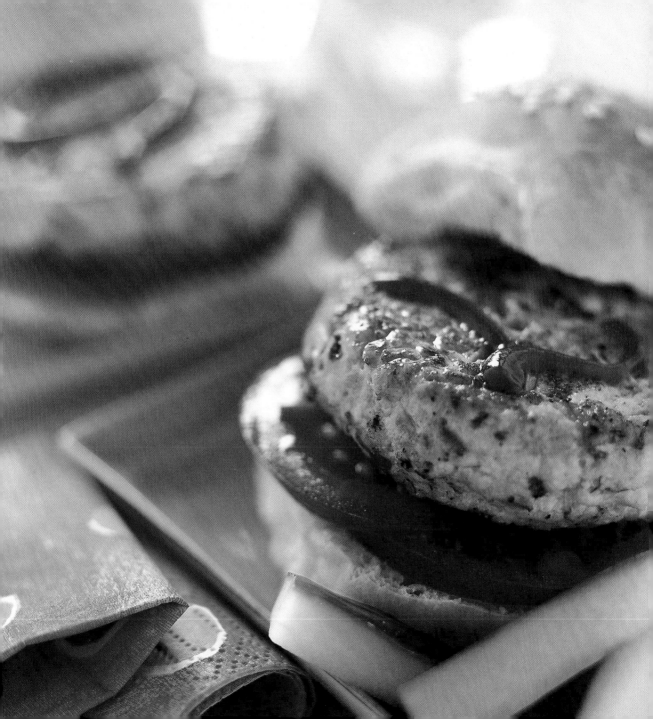

Teriyaki Beef Skewers

MAKES 4 SKEWERS

MARINADE

3 tablespoons soy sauce

¼ cup mirin (sweet rice wine)

1 tablespoon sesame oil

1 clove garlic, crushed

½ teaspoon grated fresh
  gingerroot

10 ounces round steak, cut
  into cubes

1 teaspoon cornstarch

A quick, easy, and delicious meal is made by marinating beef in a tasty combination of flavors and then cooking the beef on skewers for 3 to 4 minutes each side. Not only does marinating make the meat really tasty, it also makes it much more tender.

Combine all the ingredients for the marinade and marinate the cubes of beef for at least 1 hour. Soak four bamboo skewers in water while the beef is marinating. Before cooking, strain and reserve the marinade and then thread the beef onto the skewers.

COOK THE SKEWERS, either on a barbecue or under a preheated broiler, for 3 to 4 minutes each side. Meanwhile, mix the cornstarch to a paste with 1 tablespoon of the marinade, then pour into a small pan together with the remaining marinade. Bring to a boil and then simmer, stirring until thickened. This will make a delicious dipping sauce.

Annabel's Tasty Chicken Skewers

These skewers can be interspersed with some vegetables such as chunks of red bell pepper, onion, or button mushrooms. Brush the vegetables with the marinade before cooking the skewers. Alternatively, make skewers with chicken only and serve with boiled rice. Stir-fry chopped onion and diced red and yellow bell peppers in some olive oil and stir into the cooked rice to give it both color and flavor. This marinade is also good for salmon.

Put the soy sauce and sugar into a small saucepan and gently heat, stirring, until the sugar has dissolved. Remove from the heat, stir in the lime juice, oil, garlic, and ginger, if using. Marinate the chicken for at least 1 hour or overnight. Soak eight bamboo skewers in water to prevent them from getting scorched. Preheat the oven to 350°F. Thread the chunks of chicken onto the skewers and bake in the oven for 4 to 5 minutes on each side, basting occasionally with the marinade until cooked through. Or grill on the barbecue.

MAKES 8 SKEWERS

MARINADE

¼ cup soy sauce

⅓ cup light brown sugar

1 tablespoon lime or lemon juice

1 tablespoon canola oil

1 clove garlic, crushed

¼ teaspoon grated fresh gingerroot (optional)

4 boneless, skinless chicken breasts, cut into chunks

OVERLEAF: Corn on the Cob (page 155), Honey and Soy Salmon Skewers (page 162), Georgia Peaches (page 163), Annabel's Tasty Chicken Skewers (this page)

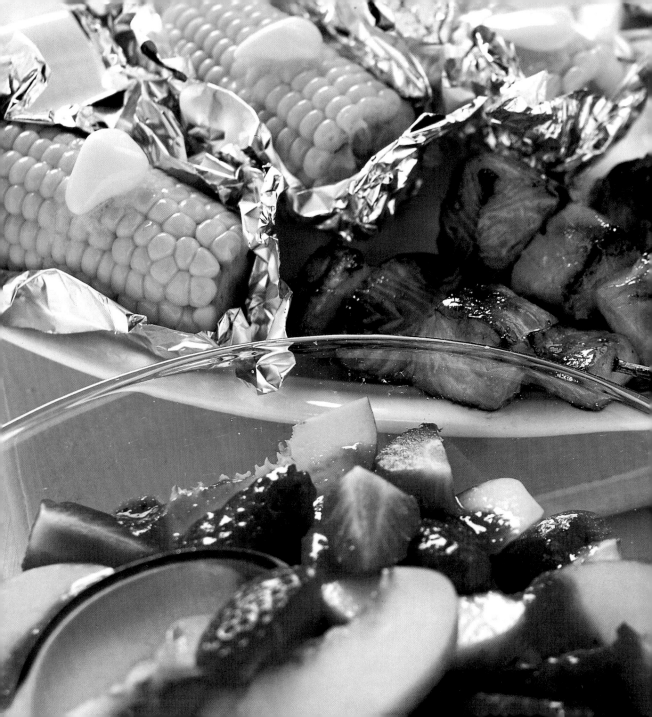

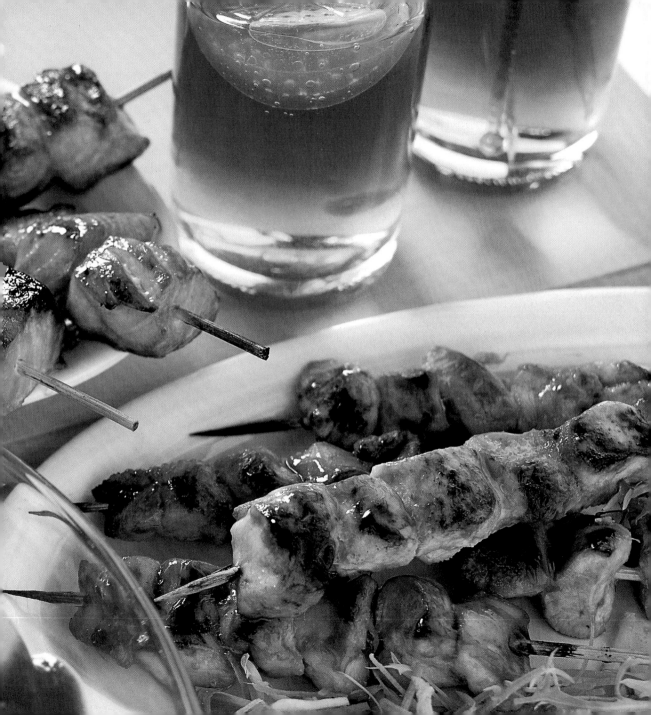

Honey and Soy Salmon Skewers

This is a delicious way to cook salmon that keeps the fish really moist and tasty.

MARINADE

1 tablespoon sesame oil

1 tablespoon soy sauce

1 tablespoon honey

One 12- to 14-ounce salmon
    fillet, skinned and cut into
    1½-inch cubes

Mix together the sesame oil, soy sauce, and honey. Marinate the cubes of salmon in this mixture for at least 30 minutes. Meanwhile, soak four bamboo skewers in water to prevent them from getting scorched. Thread the cubes of salmon onto the skewers and barbecue over medium-hot coals for 2 to 3 minutes, turning occasionally and basting with the remaining marinade until golden on the outside but still moist and juicy in the center.

ALTERNATIVELY, preheat the broiler. Remove the salmon from the marinade, line a baking pan with foil, and arrange the cubes of salmon on the foil. Broil for 8 minutes, turning halfway through the cooking time and basting with the remaining marinade.

Georgia Peaches

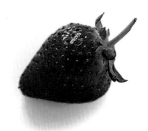

This is a delicious, quick, and easy dessert to make when berries and peaches are in season. The sauce could also be poured over strawberries and blueberries.

SERVES 4

1½ cups raspberries, fresh or
  frozen
2 tablespoons confectioners'
  sugar
1 cup strawberries
2 ripe peaches, peeled and
  sliced
4 scoops vanilla ice cream
  (optional)

If using frozen raspberries, heat them in a saucepan until mushy. If using fresh raspberries, puree them in a food processor. Press the raspberries through a nylon strainer to remove the seeds, then stir in the sugar. Halve or quarter the strawberries according to their size and mix with the sliced peaches. Divide the fruit among four serving dishes and pour the raspberry sauce on top. Top with ice cream, if desired.

Luscious Lychee Ice Pops

This is a real winner for a hot summer day.

MAKES 4 LARGE OR 6 SMALL
  ICE POPS

One 20-ounce can lychees
1 tablespoon lemon juice

Puree the lychees with the syrup from the can and strain. Stir in the lemon juice and pour into ice pop molds. Freeze.

Halloween

You will need: white handkerchiefs, black felt-tip pen, lollipops, tissue paper, black ribbon or elastic bands, padded envelopes.

Keeping the centers white, write the party details around the edges of the handkerchiefs using the black felt-tip pen. Place the centers of two sheets of tissue paper over each lollipop. Put a handkerchief on top of each and, where the lollipop meets the stick, fasten with the ribbon or use an elastic band. With the black felt-tip pen, draw two eyes on the ghost's face. Send out the invitations to your guests in a padded envelope, decorated with Halloween stickers if you like.

Halloween is a wonderful opportunity to dress up, and these costumes are really easy to make. For example, create a ghost from an old white sheet with two holes cut out for eyes and outlined with black felt-tip pen, or make a mummy by wrapping a child in toilet paper secured with masking tape. For a witch's costume, use black oak tag for a hat and a black plastic trash bag with the hem cut into zigzags for a dress; add hair made from strips of a green plastic trash bag or use some green yarn.

Adding to the Fun

- There are loads of wonderful accessories you can buy at costume shops, such as battery-operated headgear with flashing pumpkins or devil's horns; gnarled, luminous witches' fingers; or fangs and fake blood.
- If you want children to come trick-or-treating at your door, carve out a pumpkin and place a lit candle inside.

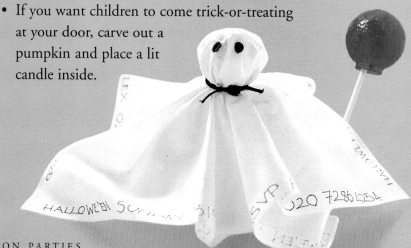

Halloween Games

Apple Bobbing

Props: large bowl, apples, old newspapers.
Half fill a bowl with water and float apples
on top. Taking turns, the children have to
lift an apple out of the water using only
their teeth while keeping their hands behind
their backs. Children can wear aprons if you
have them. Spread plenty of newspaper over
the floor, as this can get quite messy!

Witch's Cauldron

Props: large bowl, cloth to cover bowl,
paper, pencils.
Suggested contents: hairy toy spider,
marshmallow, tea bag, bar of soap, tooth
brush, tennis ball, clementine, avocado, emery
board, Milky Way bar, wine bottle cork.

Place about ten objects in the "cauldron,"
turn off the lights, and cover it up with a
cloth. Let each child in turn feel the
contents, leave the room, and write down
what they are. All the lists are given to an
adult who reads out the children's guesses.
The one who guesses the most objects
correctly is the winner.

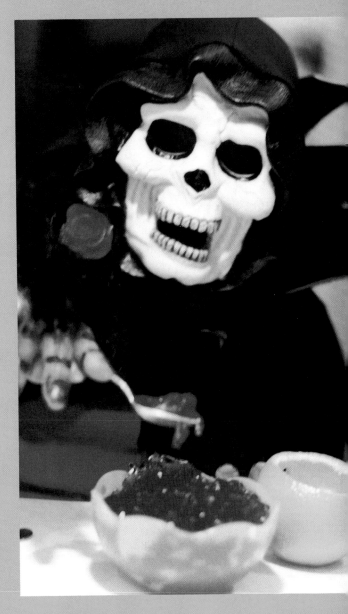

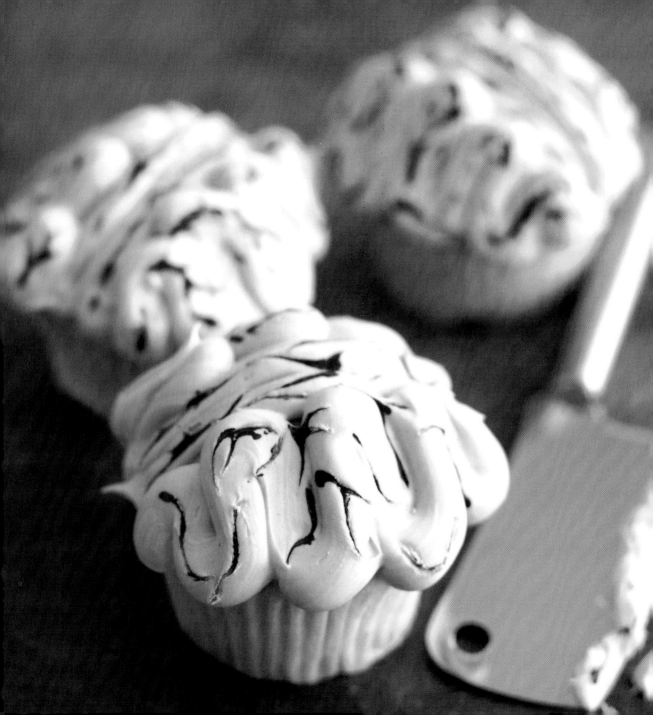

Brain Cupcakes

Making cupcakes that look like brains is fun for Halloween.

Add confectioners' sugar to creamy vanilla frosting to make it stiff enough to pipe. Add a little red and black food coloring to make the "brain" pinkish gray. Pipe the frosting on top of cupcakes (use a cake mix, your favorite recipe, or see pages 169 and 170) and, using red food coloring and a toothpick, draw red veins on the icing. Serve up the cupcakes and play this game:

Body Parts

Only the bravest should get involved in this game. The idea is for the players to plunge their hands into bowls of nasty things they can't see and guess what they are. This is a vey spooky touchy-feely game that will send shivers down your spine.

Have several bowls and cover each one with a cloth so that the children can't see what is inside. Here are some suggestions:

- Peeled grapes for eyeballs
- Cooked, cooled linked sausages for intestines
- Cooked cauliflower for brains
- Balloon filled with water for a heart
- Wet cooked spaghetti for veins
- Gelatin for liver

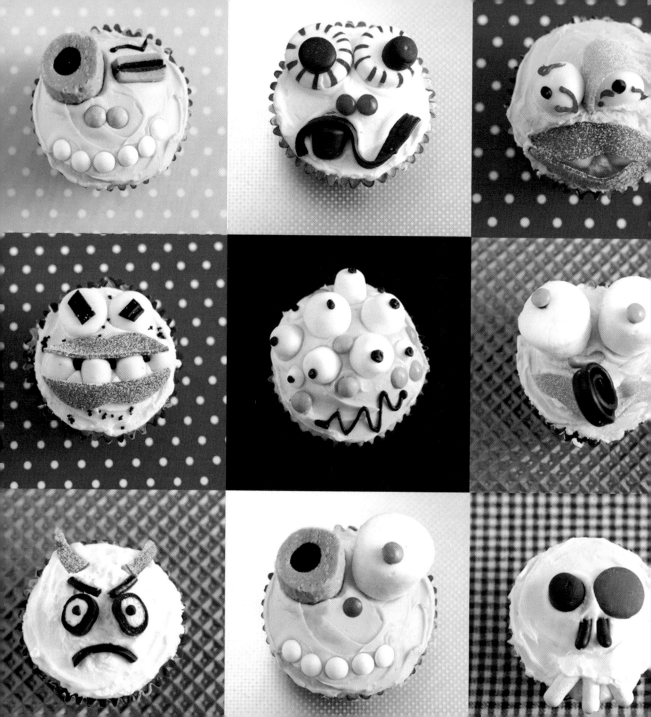

Eyeball Cupcakes

Sweet food normally looks so mouthwatering—but not these scary treats! Let your guests eat them if they dare. Use my ideas for inspiration, then create your own eyeball cupcakes.

Preheat the oven to 350°F and line two muffin pans with 20 paper liners. Sift together the flour, baking powder, and salt. In an electric mixer, beat the butter. Gradually beat in the sugar until light and fluffy. Add the eggs one at a time, beating between each addition. Pour the milk into a measuring cup and add the vanilla.

Add about a quarter of the flour mixture to the butter and beat well. Add about a quarter of the milk and vanilla and mix well. Continue alternately adding flour and then milk, beating well after each addition, until the mixture is smooth. Fill the liners about three-quarters full.

Bake for about 20 minutes. You can tell when the cupcakes are done when they have risen, are golden in color, and spring back when pressed. Remove the cupcakes from the oven, allow to cool for a few minutes, and then turn them out of the pan and onto a wire rack to cool completely.

When cool, spread half the cupcakes with white frosting and half with frosting that you've tinted green. Create eyes, noses, and mouths using the candies and writing icing.

MAKES 20 CUPCAKES

3 cups all-purpose flour

1½ teaspoons baking powder

½ teaspoon salt

1 stick plus 2 tablespoons unsalted butter, softened

1¾ cups superfine sugar

2 large eggs

1¼ cups milk

1 teaspoon pure vanilla extract

DECORATION

One 16-ounce tub vanilla frosting (Betty Crocker Rich & Creamy Frosting)

Green food coloring

Assorted candies

Tubes writing icing

Green Monster Cupcakes

MAKES 12 CUPCAKES

You can have fun with your children designing ghoulish cupcakes for Halloween.

1 cup self-rising flour

1 stick unsalted butter, softened

⅔ cup superfine sugar

2 large eggs

1 teaspoon pure vanilla extract

DECORATION

One 16-ounce tub vanilla frosting (Betty Crocker Rich & Creamy Frosting)

Green food coloring

Marshmallows (regular and mini)

Strawberry licorice laces

Licorice Allsorts

Gummy rings

Gumdrops

Candy-coated chocolate

Fruit leather

Sour tape

Nonpareils

Preheat the oven to 350°F. Put all the cupcake ingredients in a bowl and beat together until the mixture is smooth and creamy. Line a muffin pan with paper liners and fill each half full with batter. You can also make mini cupcakes (see recipe for Stars and Stripes Mini Cupcakes, page 153).

Bake for 18 to 20 minutes. You can tell when the cupcakes are done when they have risen, are golden in color, and spring back when pressed. Remove the cupcakes from the oven, allow to cool for a few minutes, and then turn them out of the pan and onto a wire rack to cool completely.

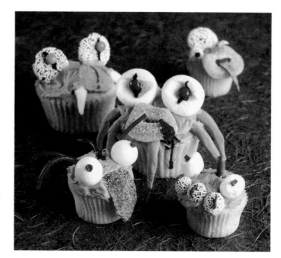

TINT THE FROSTING green with food coloring. Spread the frosting over the tops of the cupcakes and decorate.

Meatballs with Sweet-and-Sour Sauce

On a cold autumn night it is nice to give the children a warming supper after trick-or-treating. This recipe is ideal; it is delicious and very popular with my three children, and it can be made in advance and frozen if you wish. Serve with rice.

Finely crumble the bouillon cube and then mix together all the ingredients for the meatballs except the oil and chop for a few seconds in a food processor together with 2 tablespoons cold water. Using floured hands, form into about 20 meatballs. Heat the oil in a frying pan and sauté the meatballs, turning occasionally, for 10 to 12 minutes until browned.

FOR THE SAUCE, mix together the soy sauce and cornstarch. Heat the oil in a pan and sauté the onion for 3 minutes. Add the bell pepper and sauté for 2 minutes, stirring occasionally. Add the tomatoes, vinegar, and sugar, season with black pepper, and simmer for 10 minutes. Add the soy sauce mixture and cook for 2 minutes, stirring occasionally. If you want a smooth sauce, you can blend or use a food mill. Pour the sauce over the meatballs, cover, and simmer for about 5 minutes.

SERVES 4 OR 5

❄

MEATBALLS

1 chicken bouillon cube

1 pound lean ground beef

1 onion, finely chopped

1 apple, peeled, grated, and squeezed to drain

½ cup fresh white bread crumbs

1 tablespoon chopped fresh parsley

Salt and freshly ground black pepper

2 tablespoons canola oil

1 tablespoon soy sauce

1½ teaspoons cornstarch

1 tablespoon canola oil

1 onion, finely chopped

¼ cup diced red bell pepper

One 14.5-ounce can chopped tomatoes

1 tablespoon malt vinegar

1 teaspoon light brown sugar

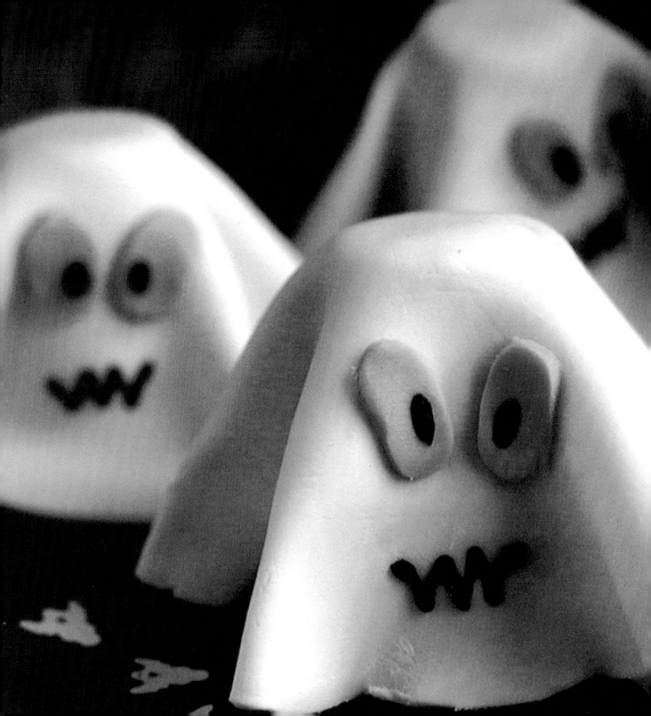

Ghoulish Ghost Cakes

Timbale molds are the ideal shape for these spooky little cakes, but you could cheat and use Ho Hos or Yodels under the white icing.

Beat together the butter, sugar, and vanilla until light and fluffy. Add the eggs one at a time, adding 1 tablespoon flour with each egg. Beat well and fold in the remaining flour. Preheat the oven to 350°F. Spoon the batter into eight greased timbale molds, place the filled molds on a baking tray, and bake for 20 minutes. Let cool, cut off the tops of the cakes to form flat surfaces, then turn out onto a board or plate. Allow to cool completely.

DUST YOUR WORK SURFACE with cornstarch and roll out the icing. Using a saucer as a guide, cut out eight 6-inch circles. Drape these over the sponge cakes to form ghosts. Color one-quarter of the remaining icing pink and make eyes. Attach with a little writing icing, then use the writing icing to draw mouths and pupils.

MAKES 8 INDIVIDUAL GHOST CAKES

❄ sponge cake only

1¾ sticks unsalted butter, plus extra for greasing

¾ cup plus 1 tablespoon superfine sugar

1 tablespoon pure vanilla extract

3 large eggs

1¼ cups self-rising flour

Cornstarch, for dusting

2 pounds white rolled fondant icing

Red food coloring

1 tube black writing icing

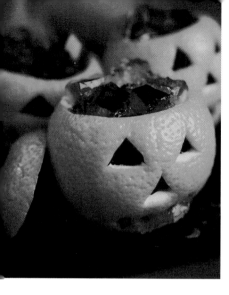

Pumpkin Oranges

These oranges are cut to look like mini pumpkins and then filled with a selection of cut-up fruits or chopped gelatin.

Cut a slice from the stem end of each orange and cut a small sliver from the base so that it stands upright. Hollow out using a small sharp knife and a teaspoon. Cut out eyes, nose, and mouth shapes from the shell.

Witches' Broomsticks

MAKES 6 BROOMSTICKS

Pretzel sticks
6 cheese straw twists
6 chives or scallion strips

These look very authentic. To make it easier to tie the chives or scallion strips, you may need to heat them in a microwave oven for 10 seconds to make them more pliable.

To assemble the broomsticks, attach pretzels onto the end of each cheese straw twist by tying them on with a knotted chive or scallion strip.

Dead Man's Fingers

These ghoulish sandwiches look terrific!

Gently flatten the slices of bread with a rolling pin to make them more pliable. Spread with a little margarine and either some cream cheese or peanut butter. Roll up the sandwiches and make three indentations with a blunt knife to form the finger joints. Stick an almond onto each tip with a little cream cheese or peanut butter to form the nails and add some strawberry jam or ketchup for the blood!

 N

Thin-sliced white bread, crusts
  removed
Soft margarine
Cream cheese or peanut
  butter
Almonds
Strawberry jam or ketchup

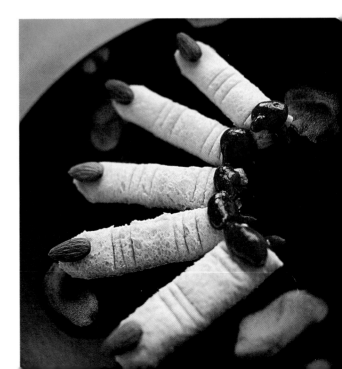

Spider and Bat Cupcakes

MAKES 10 TO 12 CUPCAKES

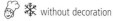 without decoration

1 stick unsalted butter or
   ½ cup soft margarine
½ cup superfine sugar
2 large eggs
¾ cup self-rising flour
   (substitute 2 tablespoons
   Dutch-process cocoa
   powder for 2 tablespoons
   of the flour for chocolate
   cupcakes)
½ teaspoon grated orange
   zest (optional)

SPIDERS
4 ounces dark or milk
   chocolate
Licorice laces
10 Mallomars
Licorice Allsorts
Mini M&M's

*To make chocolate cupcakes, simply substitute
2 tablespoons of cocoa powder for 2 teaspoons of flour.*

Preheat the oven to 350°F. Beat together the butter and sugar
until light and fluffy. Beat the eggs into the mixture one at a
time, adding a spoonful of the flour with the second egg. Sift the
flour or flour and cocoa mix (if you want chocolate cupcakes)
into the bowl and stir until well blended. If using orange zest,
add it now.

   Line a muffin pan with paper liners and spoon the batter
into the liners until about two-thirds full for the spider
cupcakes. If you want a rounded top for the bats' wings, fill
the liners a little more (this mixture will make 12 spiders but
probably 10 bats). Bake the cupcakes for 18 to 20 minutes.
Put on a wire rack to cool.

SPIDER CUPCAKES Melt the chocolate in a heatproof bowl
over a pan of simmering water. Using a spatula, cover each
cupcake with some of the melted chocolate, arrange eight laces
for the spider's legs, and stick a Mallomar in the center. Finish
with the licorice candies and M&M's for eyes.

BAT CUPCAKES To make the chocolate icing, beat the butter until creamy. Sift together the sugar and cocoa and gradually beat into the butter together with the milk using a wooden spoon. When the cupcakes have cooled, cut off the tops, cut each into three sections, and use the two curved ends to make wings (reserve the middle section).

Draw a V with black writing icing on the wings. Spread a thick layer of chocolate icing over the top of the cupcake and position the wings so that they stand up (you will need to cut small squares of cake from the middle section to position under the wings to prop them up). Stick silver balls on top of black licorice candies for the bats' eyes.

BATS

1 stick softened unsalted butter

1 cup confectioners' sugar

2 tablespoons Dutch-process
    cocoa powder

1 tablespoon milk

Black writing icing

Licorice Allsorts

Edible silver balls

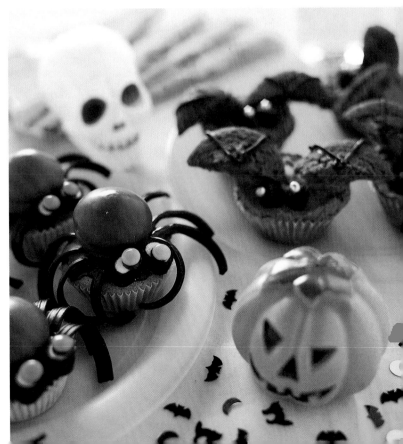

Thanksgiving

Although I'm English, I've enjoyed some lovely Thanksgiving celebrations with American friends, picking up a few helpful ideas along the way. Thanksgiving is a wonderfully festive time of year for families, and helping your children to participate in food preparation is a great way to include them in the tradition. Even simple tasks, such as mixing the dry and wet ingredients for the Corn Bread Dressing (page 180), can truly help children stay involved.

I've found that as rich and warm as the flavors of Thanksgiving are, it may take a bit of creativity to find dishes that appeal to your children. Children will hardly eat plain mashed squash, for instance. However, blend it together with a little cream, sugar, and maple syrup, as in my Creamy Maple Butternut Squash (page 182), and the children are ecstatic. They're also very pleased with the notion of marshmallows with vegetables, as in my Fluffy Marshmallow Sweet Potatoes (page 181). And to be honest, these yummy, sweet variations are always an instant hit with the parents, too.

If you'll be hosting a few small children, cutting bite-size pieces of turkey while serving the entire dinner can be a real headache. I've found that with a simple alternative like my Chicken Dippers (page 185), children stay involved and stay eating. These are popular snacks for the football-watching crew

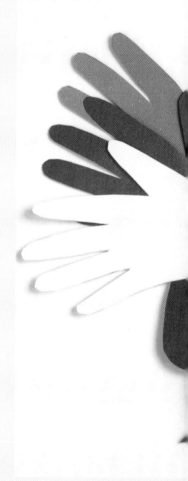

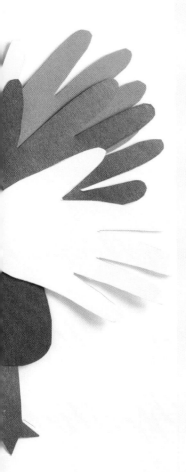

as well. I like to give the children a few dipping options—ketchup and honey—as a special holiday treat.

Consider keeping the children amused with a special Thanksgiving project, like the Hands and Feet Turkey. With all the family around, it's fun to make a whole flock of turkeys, and they look adorable on the table.

Hands and Feet Turkey

You'll need a package of colored construction paper, a pencil, scissors, some glue, and a black felt-tip pen. Using the children's hands and feet as templates, trace two feet on brown paper—older children will love to help the little ones with this part—and then trace pairs of hands onto tan, yellow, orange, and cream paper. Cut out all the hands and feet.

Put the two cutout feet together to make the turkey's body and head, spreading the heels apart, and glue them together.

Cut two turkey legs and a beak out of tan and orange paper. Cut out the wattle from red paper. Cut out eyes from white paper and draw black pupils using the felt-tip pen. Glue all these parts onto the turkey's body.

Glue the tan, yellow, and orange hands behind the turkey's body to make the tail. Glue a cream hand to each side to make the turkey's wings. Give him a name and you're done.

Corn Bread Dressing

SERVES 6

N

One 6.5-ounce package corn
    bread mix
¼ cup plus 1 tablespoon
    canola oil
¾ cup milk
2 large eggs
¼ cup plus 1 tablespoon
    freshly grated Parmesan
    cheese (optional)
2 celery stalks, chopped
1 small onion, chopped
1 clove garlic, crushed
⅓ cup dried cranberries
⅓ cup chopped pecans
2 teaspoons fresh thyme
    leaves or 1 teaspoon
    dried thyme
¾ cup chicken stock
Salt and freshly ground black
    pepper

*Serve this delicious dressing with roast turkey, gravy,
mashed potatoes, and cranberry sauce. It tastes so good
that I like to eat it on its own.*

Preheat the oven to 400°F. Put the corn bread mix into a mixing
bowl, add the ¼ cup oil, the milk, and one of the eggs, and mix
well. If you are using the Parmesan, stir ¼ cup into the batter.
Pour the batter into an 8-inch square baking pan. Bake for
20 minutes. Allow to cool and then cut into ½-inch cubes.

SAUTÉ THE CELERY, ONION, AND GARLIC very gently in the
1 tablespoon oil for about 10 minutes. Turn the oven
temperature to 350°F. Transfer the vegetables to a bowl.
Add 3 cups cubed corn bread, the cranberries, pecans, thyme,
chicken stock, and the remaining egg. Season with salt and
pepper. Put in a lightly oiled ovenproof dish. Sprinkle the
1 tablespoon Parmesan on top, if using. Bake for 30 minutes.

Fluffy Marshmallow Sweet Potatoes

This makes a delicious accompaniment to the Thanksgiving meal and it's good with or without the mini marshmallow topping.

Preheat the oven to 400°F. Wash and prick the sweet potatoes and bake for 1 hour. Allow the potatoes to cool a little. Cut in half lengthwise, scoop out the flesh, and put into a bowl. Mash together with the butter and Marshmallow Fluff. Beat in the egg and mix in the cinnamon, salt, and pepper. Transfer to a lightly buttered 9 x 13-inch baking dish. Bake for 25 minutes. Top with the mini marshmallows and bake for an additional 5 minutes.

SERVES 6

3 sweet potatoes (about 2 pounds total)

2 tablespoons unsalted butter

⅓ cup Marshmallow Fluff

1 large egg

¼ teaspoon ground cinnamon

½ teaspoon salt and a little freshly ground black pepper

1 cup mini marshmallows

Creamy Maple Butternut Squash

SERVES 8

4 large butternut squash
  (about 4 pounds total)
4 tablespoons unsalted butter,
  melted, plus extra for
  brushing the squash
¼ cup heavy cream
¼ cup maple syrup
½ teaspoon salt

Baking squash caramelizes the flavor. Delicious sweet, buttery butternut squash.

Preheat the oven to 400°F. With a sharp knife, cut the squash in half, scoop out the seeds, and brush each half generously with melted butter. Put in a baking pan, cover loosely with foil, and bake for 1 to 1½ hours until tender.

WITH A SPOON, scoop the flesh out into a bowl. If you have a food processor, puree the squash with the ¼ cup melted butter, the cream, maple syrup, and salt until smooth and creamy. Alternatively, mash it all together with a potato masher.

Strawberry and Rhubarb Crumble

This is one of my favorite crumbles. It is a delicious combination of flavors, and the pink color of the rhubarb looks so attractive. It is also very quick and easy to prepare. Serve with custard or ice cream.

Preheat the oven to 400°F. Cut the rhubarb into small pieces (not larger than ½ inch) and hull and halve the strawberries. Combine with the superfine sugar. Sprinkle the base of a suitable ovenproof dish (an 8-inch round Pyrex dish looks nice) with ¼ cup of the ground almonds. Spoon in the fruit mixture.

TO MAKE THE TOPPING, mix the flour together with the brown sugar and salt in a bowl and rub in the butter using your fingertips until the mixture resembles bread crumbs. Stir in the remaining ½ cup almonds. Cover the fruit with the crumble topping and bake for about 30 minutes.

SERVES 5

❄ **N**

1 pound rhubarb

6 strawberries

¼ cup superfine sugar

¾ cup ground almonds

CRUMBLE TOPPING

1 cup all-purpose flour

½ cup light brown sugar

Generous pinch of salt

1 stick cold unsalted butter,
    cut into pieces

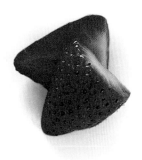

Celebration Coleslaw

Coleslaw with a twist—I have added diced red apple and raisins. It tastes so good I like to eat it all year round.

Toss the apple with the lemon juice and mix together with the coleslaw and raisins. Whisk together the mayonnaise, vinegar, and sugar with 2 teaspoons water and toss with the coleslaw mixture.

1 red apple, cored and diced (do not peel)

2 tablespoons lemon juice

Half a 1-pound package coleslaw mix (shredded cabbage and carrot)

½ cup raisins

½ cup mayonnaise

1 teaspoon white wine vinegar

2 teaspoons sugar

Annabel's Chicken Dippers

SERVES 4

- 2 boneless, skinless chicken breasts
- ¼ cup freshly grated Parmesan cheese
- ¼ cup grated Cheddar cheese
- ¼ cup dried bread crumbs
- ½ teaspoon paprika
- ¼ to ½ teaspoon cayenne pepper
- Salt and freshly ground black pepper
- 1 large egg, lightly beaten
- 2 tablespoons all-purpose flour
- ⅓ cup sunflower or other vegetable oil for frying

Some picky eaters just don't like turkey, but these are always gobbled up. (They're yummy anytime with fries, served in a rolled-up cone made from a comics page lined with waxed paper.)

Cut each chicken breast into ½-inch strips. Mix together the Parmesan, Cheddar, bread crumbs, paprika, cayenne, and salt and pepper to taste. Place the egg in a shallow dish, the flour in another, and the cheesy bread crumb mixture in a third. Dip each chicken strip first into the flour, then into the beaten egg, and finally coat with the bread crumb mixture.

Pour the oil into a frying pan and cook the chicken over medium heat in batches, taking care not to crowd the pan. Sauté for about 2 minutes on each side until golden. Drain on paper towels.

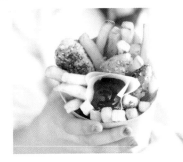

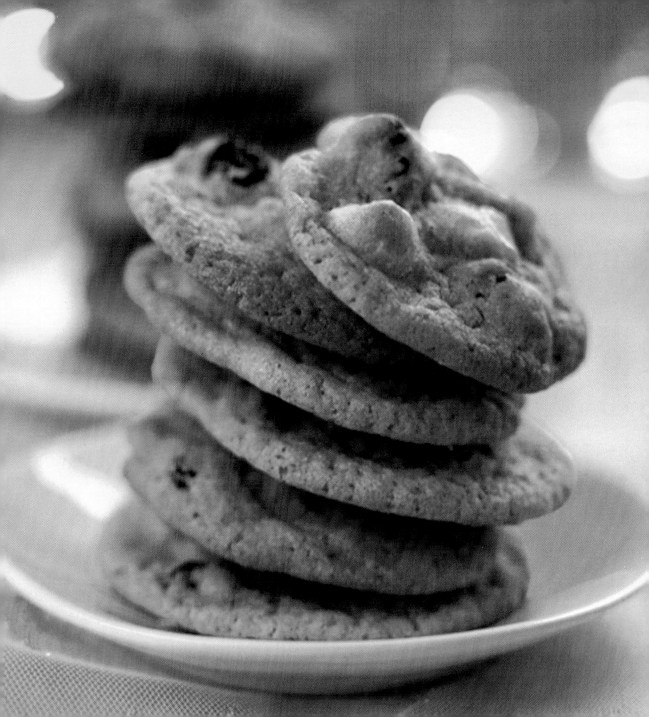

Cranberry and White Chocolate Cookies

These are not to be missed; they are probably my favorite cookies and are so quick and easy to make. You can buy dried cranberries in the supermarket.

Preheat the oven to 375°F. Sift together the flour, baking soda, and salt into a large bowl. Stir in the ground almonds, brown sugar, oats, cranberries, and white chocolate chunks. Melt the butter in a small pan. Stir into the dry ingredients together with the egg yolk. Mix well and then, using your hands, form into walnut-size balls and arrange on two large nonstick baking sheets. Gently press the balls down to flatten slightly, leaving space between them for the cookies to spread. Bake for 12 minutes, then remove and let cool on a wire rack. They will be quite soft but will firm up as they cool. I like them to have a soft, chewy center.

MAKES 20 COOKIES

N

1 cup all-purpose flour

½ teaspoon baking soda

½ teaspoon salt

¼ cup ground almonds

¾ cup light brown sugar

1 cup rolled oats

½ cup dried cranberries

2 ounces white chocolate, cut into chunks

1 stick plus 2 tablespoons unsalted butter

1 large egg yolk or 2 small egg yolks

Christmas

CHRISTMAS CRACKER INVITATIONS
You will need: empty toilet paper tubes, white paper, gold tissue paper, shiny red paper, gold ribbon, Christmas decorations such as holly, padded envelopes.

Write the details of the party on a piece of paper and wrap it around an empty toilet paper tube. If you wish, put a little gift like a balloon or candy inside the tube. Cover with gold tissue and shiny red paper and tie the ends with gold ribbon to look like a firecracker. If you like, stick on some Christmas decorations. Send out in a padded envelope.

Christmas is a magical time of year and when the theme for a party is Christmas, it is a fantastic excuse for dressing up. Children will love to dress up as such perennial favorites as Santa Claus, angels, snowmen, Christmas trees—or even Rudolph the red-nosed reindeer.

Adding to the Fun

- Get the children involved in activities such as baking and decorating Christmas cookies. You can use the recipe for Stained-Glass Window Cookies (page 198) or Heart-Shaped Faces (page 66) and use Christmas cookie cutters such as bells, angels, stockings, and Christmas trees to shape the cookies. Put out plenty of decorating items such as colored sugar, tubes of writing icing, and sprinkles.

- It is also fun to make snowflakes from pieces of paper folded into quarters. You will need lots of pairs of scissors, pencils, crayons, and glitter. Show the children how to draw patterns on the folded paper, then cut them out so that when the paper is opened, the result is a cutout snowflake ready for coloring and decorating with glitter before hanging on the tree.

- Every year we sing Christmas songs and carols, but how well do we know them? You could play excerpts of various Christmas music and ask the children to try to write down the titles of the songs. The child with the most correct answers is the winner.

Christmas Games

Hunt the Christmas Card

Props: old Christmas cards, scissors.

Cut the fronts of the Christmas cards in half. Put one set of the halves in a basket and divide them among the children. Hide the other halves around the house and ask the children to search for as many of the matching halves as possible in a given time.

Christmas Stocking

Props: Christmas stocking, various objects.

Put various objects into a Christmas stocking without the children seeing what they are. Have a mixture of things, some more unusual than others. The children then have to feel the stocking and guess what is inside.

Pin the Nose on Rudolph

Props: blindfold, large picture of Rudolph, red nose, and thumb tack.

This is a Christmas version of pin the tail on the donkey. Every child has a go trying to pin the red nose in the correct place while blindfolded. It is a good idea to turn the children around a few times once they are blindfolded to disorient them. Mark the spot where each child places the thumb tack with an X and their initials to see who comes the closest.

Christmas Drawings

Props: paper and pencils.

Make a list of things to do with Christmas, such as reindeers, snowmen, angels. Divide the children into teams and ask the first child from each team to come up so you can whisper in their ear the name of the object. They must then go back to their team members and draw it. As soon as a team member guesses correctly, the next person goes up, and so on. To make this more difficult, ask the children to draw the object with the wrong hand.

Rudolph the Red-Nosed Baked Potato

MAKES 4 BAKED POTATOES

4 medium baking potatoes
  (about 8 ounces each)
Canola oil
½ medium butternut squash
  (about 10 ounces)
3 tablespoons unsalted butter,
  plus extra for brushing
  the squash
¼ cup freshly grated
  Parmesan cheese
1 teaspoon Dijon mustard
2 tablespoons milk
Salt and freshly ground
  black pepper
¼ cup grated Cheddar cheese

DECORATION
Cherry tomatoes
Cooked frozen peas
Cheese straw twists or
  pretzel sticks

A great recipe for turning a baked potato into a delicious mouthwatering treat for Christmas.

Preheat the oven to 375°F. Prick the potatoes in several places, place on a baking pan, and brush all over with the oil. Bake for 1 hour to 1 hour 15 minutes until they feel soft when pressed.

CUT THE BUTTERNUT SQUASH in half, scoop out the seeds, and brush with a pat of melted butter. Bake for about 40 minutes until tender.

WHEN COOL ENOUGH TO HANDLE, cut the tops off the baked potatoes and scoop out the flesh. Scoop out the flesh of the cooked butternut squash and mash together with the baked potato flesh, Parmesan, mustard, milk, and butter. Season with a little salt and pepper. Put the mixture back into the potato shells, cover with the grated Cheddar, and cook under the broiler for a few minutes or until golden.

DECORATE WITH A CHERRY TOMATO for the nose, peas for the eyes, and cheese straw twists or pretzel sticks for the antlers.

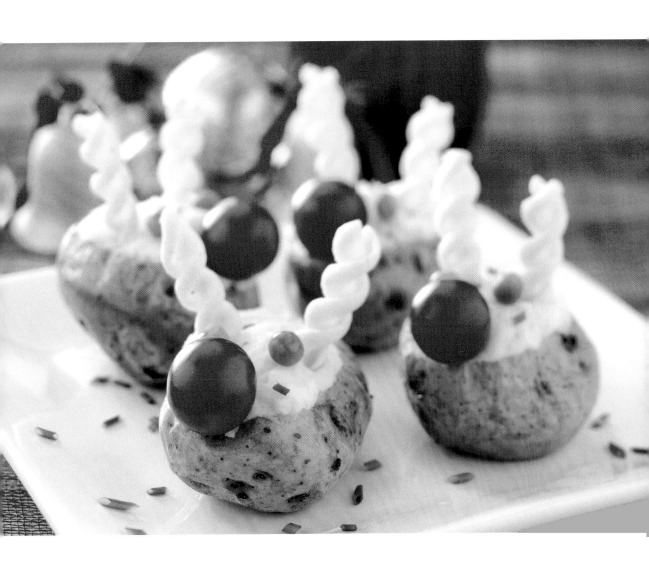

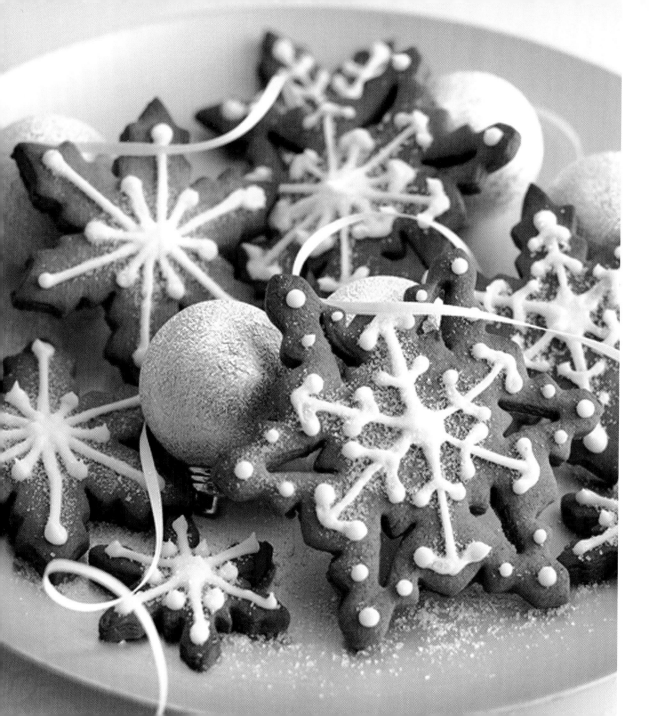

Cookie Exchange

MAKES ABOUT 24 COOKIES

1 stick plus 2 tablespoons
   butter, softened
½ cup packed light
   brown sugar
½ cup molasses
1 large egg yolk
2½ cups all-purpose flour
1 teaspoon baking soda
Pinch of salt
1 tablespoon ground ginger
1 teaspoon pumpkin pie spice

ROYAL ICING

4½ cups confectioners' sugar
5 tablespoons meringue
   powder

White decorating (sanding)
   sugar, for sprinkling

Baking cookies is a favorite holiday tradition but one that often gets pushed to the bottom of the to-do list. This year try hosting a cookie exchange and involve your children. Everyone brings one type of cookie, but each guest goes home with a whole variety of holiday treats. Buy some disposable containers to package and share the cookies when they are baked. Have your guests tell you in advance what they are baking to avoid duplication and ask them to bring enough copies of the recipe for everyone attending.

Gingerbread Snowflakes

Cream together the butter and sugar. Beat in the molasses and egg yolk. Sift in the dry ingredients to form a dough. Divide the dough in half. Mold into two balls, wrap in plastic, and chill in the fridge for about 30 minutes.

PREHEAT THE OVEN TO 400°F. Roll out the dough on a lightly floured work surface to about ¼-inch thick. Cut into snowflakes using snowflake cutters. Arrange them on baking sheets lined with parchment or other baking paper. Bake the cookies for about 10 minutes (smaller cookies will take less time). Allow to cool for a few minutes and then transfer to wire racks.

To make the royal icing, put the sugar, meringue powder, and a scant ½ cup water in the bowl of an electric mixer with the paddle attachment. Mix on low until smooth, about 7 minutes. If the icing is too thick, add a little extra water. Put the icing in a pastry bag fitted with a small plain round tip. Pipe designs on the snowflakes and immediately sprinkle with decorating sugar. Let stand for 5 minutes and tap off the excess sugar.

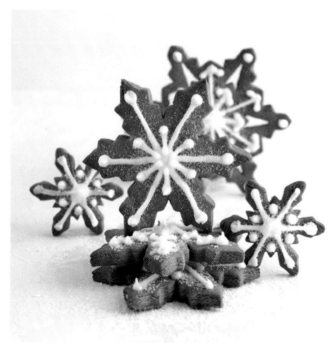

Snickerdoodles

Snickerdoodles—don't you just love the name?—are a traditional Christmas cookie in North America and are quick and easy to make. They have a characteristically crackly surface and can be crisp or soft, depending on preference. While the origin of the name has been lost, it has been speculated that "snick" may be a reference to Saint Nicholas.

MAKES 24 COOKIES

1 stick unsalted butter, softened

½ cup solid vegetable shortening

1 teaspoon pure vanilla extract

1½ cups plus 3 tablespoons sugar

2 large eggs

2¾ cups all-purpose flour

1 teaspoon baking soda

½ teaspoon salt

1½ tablespoons ground cinnamon

Mix the butter, shortening, vanilla, and 1½ cups sugar together in a mixing bowl and beat together until fluffy. Beat in the eggs one at a time. Whisk together the flour, baking soda, and salt and mix into the first mixture.

Preheat the oven to 350°F. Grease nonstick baking pans. Mix together the 3 tablespoons sugar and the cinnamon on a large plate. Roll the dough into 1-inch balls and roll in the sugar and cinnamon mix. Space 3 inches apart on the baking pans, as they will spread, and bake for 10 to 11 minutes until lightly golden.

Allow to cool, then remove from the baking pans with a spatula and arrange on wire racks to crisp. You can then dust them with a little extra sugar and cinnamon. Store in an airtight container.

Thumbprint Cookies

MAKES 26 COOKIES

1½ sticks unsalted butter, softened

¾ cup sugar

½ teaspoon salt

2 large egg yolks

¾ teaspoon pure vanilla extract

2 cups all-purpose flour

Confectioners' sugar

Seedless raspberry jam or strawberry jam

If you want cookies with deep hollows so that you can fill them with lots of jam, choose someone with a large thumb to press into the center of the cookie. It's a lot of fun to get everyone in the family involved in making these and see if you can still recognize their thumbprint once the cookies are baked.

Cream the butter and sugar together in a mixing bowl. Add the salt, egg yolks, and vanilla and beat in. Add the flour and mix to make a dough. Roll tablespoons of the dough into balls. Place about 1 inch apart on nonstick baking sheets.

Preheat the oven to 350°F. Press down the center of each ball firmly with your thumb or use the underside of a round measuring spoon to make a perfect circle. Bake for 10 to 12 minutes. Allow to cool for a few minutes, then transfer to wire racks to cool completely. Dust with confectioners' sugar and fill the hollows with ½ to 1 teaspoon of raspberry jam each.

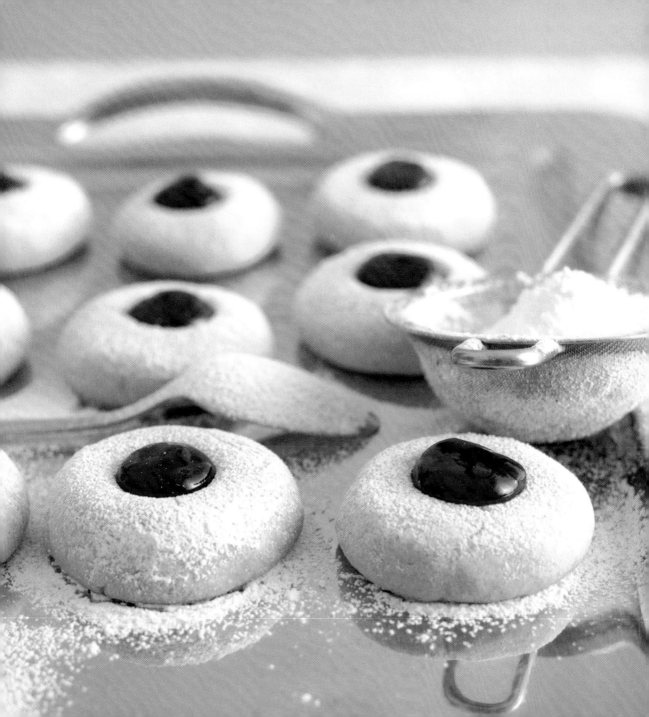

Stained-Glass Window Cookies

MAKES 25 TO 30 COOKIES

1 stick unsalted butter,
   softened

¼ cup superfine sugar

1 cup plus 2 tablespoons
   all-purpose flour

2 tablespoons cornstarch

Pinch of salt

1 teaspoon milk

18 clear hard candies, in
   assorted colors

DECORATION

1 tube white writing icing or
   Royal Icing (see page 104)

Edible silver balls

Ribbon

These novelty Christmas cookies shaped like Christmas trees, stars, bells, and snowmen are fun to make together with children and look very attractive hanging on a Christmas tree.

Preheat the oven to 350°F. Cream together the butter and sugar. Sift the flour and cornstarch together with the salt and mix together with the creamed butter and sugar. Add the milk and knead to form a soft ball of dough.

ONE COLOR AT A TIME, and using a rolling pin, crush the candies in their wrappers. Sprinkle flour on a clean work surface and roll out the dough to a thickness of about ¼ inch. Using a selection of Christmas cookie cutters, cut out shapes and arrange on baking sheets lined with parchment or other baking paper. Cut out a "window" in the center of each cookie, making sure you leave a good edge at the top and around the sides.

COMPLETELY FILL EACH CUTOUT AREA with crushed candies of one color. Make a hole at the top of each cookie using a drinking straw so that you will be able to thread a ribbon through it later.

Bake for 10 to 12 minutes until golden. While the cookies are still warm, check that the holes are still there, otherwise gently push a straw through again. Do not remove the cookies from the baking sheets until they have cooled, as the candies need to harden. Once set, gently lift the cookies off the paper with a spatula and cool on wire racks.

Decorate the cookies with white writing icing or piped royal icing and edible silver balls. Thread ribbon through the holes to make loops for hanging.

Ice Cream Snowballs

Simply roll scoops of ice cream in grated white chocolate and return to the freezer to set.

ACKNOWLEDGMENTS

To Nicolas, Lara, and Scarlett, who have been enthusiastic guinea pigs
to my triumphs and disasters; may life always be one big party.

To my mother, Evelyn Etkind, in appreciation of all the parties she gave me.

To my husband, Simon Karmel, for whom happiness is a bowl of jelly.

To Dave King and Daniel Pangbourne,
who have brought my food alive with their superb photography.

To the lovely Caroline Stearns,
who has helped me with many of the recipes in the book;
it's always a pleasure working together in the kitchen.

To Steve Linder, my alter ego in New York.

I would also like to thank Marina Magpoc, David Karmel,
Jacqui Morley, Letty Catada, Dagmar Vessely, and Janis Donnaud.

I would like to thank the team at Atria:
Judith Curr, Greer Hendricks, Hannah Morrill, Sybil Pincus,
Virginia McRae, Annette Corkey, Tess Tabor, Kathleen Schmidt, and Gary Urda.

For more information, please visit the following sites:
www.nycake.com
www.winbeckler.com
www.annabelkarmel.com

index

Annabel Karmel is a leading author on cooking for children. After the tragic loss of her first child, who died of a rare viral disease at just three months, she wrote her first book, *The Healthy Baby Meal Planner,* which is now an international bestseller. Annabel has written thirteen more bestselling books on feeding children, including *Top 100 Baby Purees, Favorite Family Meals, First Meals, and Lunchboxes.* The mother of three, she is an expert at creating tasty and nutritious meals that children like to eat without the need for parents to spend hours in the kitchen. Annabel writes regularly for national newspapers and is a familiar face on British television as an expert on children's nutritional issues. She travels frequently to the United States, where her books on feeding babies and young children are very popular, and has appeared on the *Today* show and *The Early Show.* Annabel has recently launched a "Make Your Own" line of equipment and foods to help mothers prepare fresh baby food. For more recipes and advice, visit www.annabelkarmel.com.

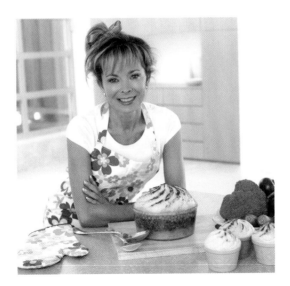

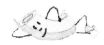
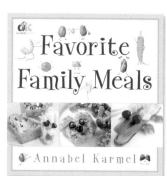
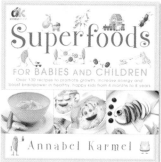
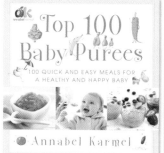
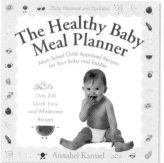